›vernment Procedures and Operations

›ing an End to Surprise Medical Billing
›al E. Tackett (Editor)
›. ISBN: 979-8-88697-296-2 (Hardcover)
›. ISBN: 979-8-88697-327-3 (eBook)

›rtion Rights, Access, and Legislative Response
›e P. Sandford (Editor)
›2. ISBN: 979-8-88697-258-0 (Softcover)
›2. ISBN: 979-8-88697-294-8 (eBook)

›iew of Capitol Police Procedures During the Capitol Attack
›ael B. Phillips (Editor)
›2. ISBN: 979-8-88697-260-3 (Hardcover)
›2. ISBN: 978-1-53617-478-6 (eBook)

›ctions in Response to the Russian Invasion of Ukraine
› Freitag (Editor)
›2. ISBN: 979-8-88697-154-5 (Hardcover)
›2. ISBN: 979-8-88697-280-1 (eBook)

›ne U.S. Postal Service Sustainable?
›issa R. Rojas (Editor)
›0. ISBN: 978-1-53618-505-8 (Hardcover)
›0. ISBN: 978-1-53618-551-5 (eBook)

›re information about this series can be found at
›s://novapublishers.com/product-category/series/government-procedures-and-
›rations/

Government Procedures and Op

snova
New York

Fred C. Wallace
Editor

COVID-19 in Nursing Homes

Impact, Transmission and Prevention

snova
New York

Library of Congress Cataloging-in-Publication Data

ISBN: 979-8-88697-673-1

Published by Nova Science Publishers, Inc. † New York

Contents

Preface

Few places have felt the devastating effects of the Coronavirus more deeply than America's nursing homes. More than 200,000 Americans living in nursing homes and other long-term care facilities have died from the Coronavirus representing 20 percent of all Coronavirus deaths in our Nation. The ferocity with which the Coronavirus swept through our Nation's nursing homes in 2020 exposed vulnerabilities that had been building for years, for too many nursing homes had inadequate staffing and poor infection control viruses well before the pandemic. These long-standing problems helped to drive outrage that exacerbated the risks for Americans who need long-term care.

Chapter 1

Examining Long-Term Care in America: The Impact of the Coronavirus in Nursing Homes*

Committee on Oversight and Reform

Wednesday, September 21, 2022

HOUSE OF REPRESENTATIVES
COMMITTEE ON OVERSIGHT AND REFORM
SELECT SUBCOMMITTEE ON THE CORONAVIRUS CRISIS
Washington, D.C.

The subcommittee met, pursuant to notice, at 2:56 p.m., in room 2154, Rayburn House Office Building, and via Zoom; Hon. James E. Clyburn [Chairman of the subcommittee] presiding.

Present: Representatives Clyburn, Maloney, Foster, Raskin, Krishnamoorthi, Scalise, Jordan, Green, Malliotakis, and Miller-Meeks.

Also present: Representative Stefanik.

Mr. CLYBURN. Good afternoon. The committee will come to order. Without objection, the chair is authorized to declare a recess of the committee at any time. I now recognize myself for an opening statement.

---

* This is an edited, reformatted and augmented version of Hearing Before the Select Subcommittee on the Coronavirus Crisis of the Committee on Oversight and Reform, House of Representatives, Serial No. 117–105, dated September 21, 2022.

In: COVID-19 in Nursing Homes
Editor: Fred C. Wallace
ISBN: 979-8-88697-673-1

Few places have felt the devastating effects of the Coronavirus more deeply than America's nursing homes. More than 200,000 Americans living in nursing homes and other long-term care facilities have died from the Coronavirus representing 20 percent of all Coronavirus deaths in our Nation.

The outside risks to nursing home residents and workers became evident in the earliest days of the crisis. The first major coronavirus outbreak in the United States occurred in the Life Care Center of Kirkland, Washington, in February 2020, where the virus infected more than two-thirds of the facility's residents and dozens of staff, resulting in the loss of nearly 40 lives.

The ferocity with which the Coronavirus swept through our Nation's nursing homes in 2020 exposed vulnerabilities that had been building for years, for too many nursing homes had inadequate staffing and poor infection control viruses well before the pandemic.

These long-standing problems helped to drive outrage that exacerbated the risks for Americans who need long-term care. Compounding these problems, Americans at greatest risk were left behind by our leaders when the virus hit our shores. The Trump administration's failure to heed early warnings left nursing homes workers and residents ill-prepared. They refused to take steps necessary to curtail the spread of the virus before vaccines were developed, leaving nursing homes without testing and personal protective equipment necessary to detect and prevent outbreaks.

New documents obtained by the select subcommittee and released today paint a devastating picture of conditions inside large for-profit nursing homes across the country during these crucial early months of the pandemic. In reports to hotlines run by nursing home chain residents, their loved ones and staff members describe the dire conditions they were experiencing during that terrible time.

At one facility in Texas, a caller reported that employees were forced to make isolation gowns out of disposable bags that were, quote, "stapled and taped together." At another home in the Mid-west, a caller stated that employees had to wear the same disposable masks for seven days in a row.

Examples of the reports we received are illustrated here. I think we all should be able to see this. Multiple reports from facilities around the country describe severe staff shortages, with one family member commenting that, and this is a quote, "criminal for there to be so few staff members present."

These new documents also shed light on the pressure that was placed on nursing home staff. An employee at the Maryland facility who was experiencing coronavirus symptoms was reportedly told that if they—that, they would be fired if they did not come to work.

At another nursing home in Colorado, a manager pressured employees to come to work even if they feel bad and have concerns that they may be sick with COVID–19.

Fortunately, our Nation has come a long way since these dark days. Life-saving vaccines and treatments have helped to save countless lives among nursing home residents and staff. The Biden/Harris administration has prioritized protecting the health of Americans in long-term care facilities. In addition to conducting an historic vaccination campaign and dramatically increasing the supply of tests and PPE, the administration has sought to institute important reforms, such as minimum staffing requirements and measures to reduce crowding inside nursing homes.

While the heightened risks that existed in 2020 have passed, risks to nursing home residents and staff will remain. We must take further steps to address long-standing challenges in this industry. We must increase the uptick of boosters among residents and staff to make sure that they stay protected against new coronavirus variants.

We must ensure that nursing home workers receive adequate pay and benefits, such as paid sick leave, which is crucial for the health and safety of residents as it is for staff.

We must also improve oversight and transparency in the nursing home industry to give residents and their loved ones the ability to make informed decisions about their care. I would like to thank all our witnesses for testifying today. I look forward to hearing more about the challenges facing our Nation's nursing homes and the changes that are needed to fix these long-standing problems so that our Nation's nursing homes are safe places for those who need care.

Before yielding to the ranking member, I ask unanimous consent that Representative Stefanik be allowed to participate in today's hearings.

Without objection, so ordered.

I now recognize the ranking member for his opening statement.

Mr. SCALISE. Thank you, Mr. Chairman. Appreciate you having this hearing, and thank you for the unanimous consent request to allow Ms. Stefanik to participate as well.

I really want to thank our witnesses for coming, and we look forward to hearing your testimony as well.

I'll keep my remarks brief to allow for a short Video that I'll be playing from Ms. Janice Dean. She and her family were affected in the worst way by the deadly nursing home policies that were put in place by a handful of Governors at the beginning of this pandemic. She's been very outspoken in talking about and trying to highlight this issue. She obviously got some very emotional feelings about this that she'll share.

It is incredibly sad, though, that what we've seen in this past year plus is a refusal to acknowledge the deadly mistakes that were made and subsequently covered up by certain Governors in nursing homes. We've highlighted this over and over again. We've called for hearings on what happened to get more transparency. We still, to this day, can't get some of that information. But we've seen thousands, tens of thousands of preventable deaths that happened because some Governors gave orders. We've highlighted these mandates over and over again by specifically five Governors who seemed to all, almost cookie cutter, take the same order over and over again to go against science, to go against the CDC and the CMS guidance for how to properly take care of nursing home patients in a nursing home setting.

If you go back to when the Trump administration wrote numerous documents to protect the elderly, to protect the vulnerable, especially in nursing homes, and I've included some comments from CDC from CMS, where they talked about things like limiting visitors, increasing protective equipment, and strengthening the quarantine guidelines in nursing homes, especially.

Clearly, some of the states that I referenced ignored that went against the science. Despite the cover-ups that we've seen, here's what we do know: Completely ignoring the CDC and CMS scientific recommendations that positive patients not be admitted back into nursing homes without the availability of proper care, multiple Governors mandated that COVID-positive patients, in fact, be admitted or readmitted to the nursing home setting, despite the fact, in some cases, that they knew they were COVID positive.

In fact, if you read the Governor of New York's mandate—and again, the state of New York, like in most states, the state is the regulator of nursing homes. I'll just read from the advisory. March 25, 2020, Mandate from New York to all nursing homes, quote: No resident shall be denied readmission or admission to the nursing home solely based on a confirmed or suspected diagnosis of COVID–19. Nursing homes are prohibited from requiring a hospitalized resident who is determined medically stable to be tested for COVID–19 prior to admission or readmission.

Again, going against the science that CMS and CDC laid out. The regulator, not just New York, but then it was almost cookie cutter, cut and pasted by the Governor of New Jersey, we saw the Governor of Michigan do the same thing, the Governor of Pennsylvania, and the Governor of California all gave mandates very similarly saying that you had to, as a nursing home, take patients back even if they were COVID positive and prohibited them from testing for COVID. And should anybody be shocked of the results we saw? Tens of thousands of patients died who never should have died.

These orders were in direct conflict with the science. We saw it with Governor Cuomo. He actively and multiple times covered up the total number of COVID–19 nursing home deaths by not reporting those nursing home residents that died in hospitals. Governor Cuomo and his team engaged in a cover-up that was designed to deceive the public and protect the Governor's image and personal profits from a multi-million-dollar book deal. He had millions of reasons to cover up the truth.

No wonder Governor Cuomo refused our request to testify. We asked him to testify at this very hearing, and he still, to this day, has not even responded. Surely, he's not here, he's not participating, but he didn't even feel he owed those victims a response to the questions we had for him.

I continue to be shocked that my colleagues on the other side of the aisle have largely ignored this scandal. Why is excessive and preventable death in nursing homes being made a partisan political issue? The Democrat majority has consistently used this pandemic as a political tool to divide Americans, and it has caused great harm and led to more distrust in public health.

With that, Mr. Chairman, I would like to show the Video from Ms. Janice Dean because it does give some more insight into what happened.

Specifically, if we could run that.

[Video shown.]

Mr. SCALISE. Thank you, Mr. Chairman. Thank you, Ms. Dean, and my thoughts and prayers continue to be with Ms. Dean, with all the other family members who had loved ones who were lost during that period. We will continue, Mr. Chairman, to press for the answers.

Why were these orders by the regulators of those nursing homes sent out, mandating that they do something that went against the very science that was coming out from CDC and CMS explaining in detail how to keep seniors safe when we knew the data was there showing this is how to keep seniors safe?

They went the opposite direction and forced those nursing homes to take COVID-positive patients, banning them from testing the people that were coming back into the homes. Tens of thousands of people died unnecessarily. We will continue pressing for those answers.

With that, I yield back the balance of my time.

Mr. CLYBURN. Thank you, Mr. Scalise.

I would like to welcome today's witnesses. Dr. Alice Bonner has been a nurse practitioner caring for older adults and their families for over 30 years. Dr. Bonner is currently the senior adviser for aging at the Institute for Healthcare Improvement, the chair of the Moving Forward Nursing Home Quality Coalition, and an adjunct faculty member at the Johns Hopkins University School of Nursing.

Dr. David Grabowski is a professor of healthcare policy at Harvard Medical School, where he studies long-term care and post-acute care. He's a current member of the Medicare Payment Advisory Commission and previously served on the CMS Nursing Home Coronavirus Commission. Dr. Grabowski has appeared before Congress numerous times in the past, including at a briefing of the select subcommittee in June 2020.

Ms. Adelina Ramos is a certified nursing assistant who has worked in nursing homes for 11 years. As a staff member at the Greenville Nursing Center in Greenville, Rhode Island, she worked on the front lines of the pandemic, including periodically providing care for dozens of critical ill patients during the early months of the coronavirus pandemic.

Dr. Jasmine Travers is an assistant professor of nursing at NYU Rory Meyers College of Nursing. Her current work focuses on mitigating health disparities in long-term care for older adults. Dr. Travers is a primary care nurse practitioner and has published widely on the topics of aging, long-term care, health disparities, and work force diversity.

Mr. Daniel Arbeeny is the principal at the executive search firm CMF Partners. Mr. Arbeeny's father, Norman, passed away during the early months of the pandemic while living in a nursing home. Mr. Arbeeny, please accept our sincere condolences for your loss.

Will the witnesses please rise and raise your right hands.

Do you swear or affirm that the testimony you are about to give is the truth, the whole truth, and nothing but the truth so help you, God?

You may be seated.

Let the record show that the witnesses answered in the affirmative.

Without objection, your written statements will be made part of the record.

Dr. Bonner, you are recognized for five minutes for your opening statement.

Statement of Dr. Alice Bonner, Senior Advisor for Aging, Chair, Institute for Healthcare Improvement, Moving Forward Nursing Home Quality Coalition

Ms. BONNER. Chairman Clyburn, Ranking Member Scalise, members of the House Select Subcommittee on the Coronavirus, Representative Stefanik, and others, thank you for the opportunity to speak today on behalf of the Moving Forward Nursing Home Quality Coalition. We are a growing coalition of more than 200 action-oriented leaders and organizations that have come together this year to create action plans for effective and sustainable improvements that will be delivered in the near future. I'm here today because each and every one of us cares deeply and is committed to improving the quality of life for individuals living in nursing homes in the United States.

We have submitted a letter to the subcommittee on behalf of the coalition that outlines six ways that Congress can begin taking meaningful steps to improve nursing home quality. It's not an all-inclusive list, and not all the proposals can be done right away. Some will require more time.

We urge Congress to work alongside us to take action so that all nursing home residents receive the care and support they deserve. Nearly 1.3 million people live in our Nation's 15,000-plus nursing homes, as you know, and another 1.5 million work in them.

The coronavirus pandemic has brought an intensified sense of urgency to addressing long-standing issues of inadequate care and support. The Moving Forward Coalition is committed to improving quality by building on strong research, clinical expertise, tested models, and advocacy for sustainable improvements.

The Moving Forward Coalition's approach is different from some other groups. Our purpose is to develop, test, and promote a set of step-by-step action plans that can be implemented based on the recommendations in the National Academies of Sciences, Engineering, and Medicine report that was released in April 2022.

The coalition began this past July and has established seven committees, each focused on key priorities. Over 200 individuals and organizations, including nursing home residents, workers, policymakers, advocates, and others, have joined the coalition in just a few months. And that number continues to grow every week.

NASEM report recommendations are well-aligned with critical needs described in the White House's February 2022 fact sheet on protecting seniors and people with disabilities. Both documents clearly convey a sense of urgency to address growing gaps in care and support that were brought into sharp focus during the pandemic, as well as they cite best practices.

Every person deserves safe, high-quality, age-friendly care and support throughout their life, and the people who dedicate their professional lives to that work for whom it is a calling or the work I was meant to do, they also need the resources, compensation, training, and support to deliver that care.

I began my professional working with older adults when I was 19 years old and got a job as a nurse's aide in a nursing home when I was still in college. I proudly wear the name badge that says nurse's aide because that experience led me to a lifelong career in nursing homes because I was inspired by what was possible and what the nurses and nursing assistants did to create a positive, supportive, loving home.

I've seen how hard many nursing home teams work to provide quality care and support for older people, often under challenges such as COVID. However, I've also been in nursing homes in which care falls short of meeting basic human needs, such as getting help to go to the bathroom or getting a bath or a shower, even once a week.

Over 85 percent of nursing home residents need assistance with one or more activities of daily living, and yet many of them are not receiving that care consistently. That must change and must change as soon as possible.

While we have Federal and state regulations designed to set standards for nursing home quality, those regulations may not be fully enforced in all cases by inspectors or state surveyors. We need a regulatory framework that reinforces and rewards quality. We need to ensure that what matters to residents is part of the culture in every nursing home. All nursing homes need to be quality homes.

The Moving Forward Coalition is off to a strong start. Our committees are holding their first calls or meetings this month, and we look forward to sharing action plans with this subcommittee back in early 2023 on the work that's beginning now.

Nursing homes are a part of the healthcare system that's often overlooked. The Moving Forward Coalition is bringing individuals and organizations together to raise expectations about what is possible. We urge Congress to lead the way toward a future of nursing homes full of the humanity and grace that all of us want and deserve.

We offer the Moving Forward Coalition as a leader eager to work with Congress, state and Federal agencies, and others to improve nursing home quality now and in the future. Thank you very much for this opportunity.

Mr. CLYBURN. Thank you, Dr. Bonner.

We'll now hear from Dr. Grabowski. You are now recognized for five minutes.

Statement of Dr. David Grabowski, Professor of Health Care Policy, Department of Health Care Policy, Harvard Medical School

Mr. GRABOWSKI. Great. Thank you. Chairman Clyburn, Ranking Member Scalise, and distinguished members of the House Select Subcommittee on the Coronavirus Crisis thank you for the opportunity to testify today on this important topic.

I am here today speaking in my capacity as a professor of healthcare policy at Harvard Medical School who has studied nursing home quality for 25 years.

Residents, their families, and their caregivers have long-known that U.S. nursing home care is broken, yet this issue has gone largely unnoticed in the broader population. COVID changed this. As one family member recently stated, the pandemic has lifted the veil on what has been an invisible social ill for decades.

COVID completely devastated nursing homes in the U.S. There have been over 1.2 million COVID cases among residents leading to roughly 172,000 COVID-related fatalities. Over 2,600 nursing home staff members have died from COVID, making nursing home worker the most dangerous job in America.

Not surprisingly, both resident census and staff employment levels are still down by over 10 percent relative to their pre-pandemic levels.

A key question in directing policy resources is determining what factors were associated with COVID outbreaks in nursing homes. In a systematic review of 36 peer-reviewed studies, our research team concluded that COVID outbreaks were largely a function of where you were located versus who you were as a facility.

This does not suggest there was nothing that could have been done to prevent COVID outbreaks; rather, it suggests that policy-makers needed to adopt a system-level approach to address this problem.

It is not too late. There are several short-run and long-run reforms that can support nursing home residents and their care-givers. In the short-term, I would encourage policymakers to focus on two areas: increasing vaccination levels and improving staffing.

First, it is time to extend the initial Federal vaccine mandate for nursing home staff to include booster doses. Roughly half of all staff are not fully vaccinated; second, to ensure all residents and staff have access to a vaccine clinic, I would recommend federally supported clinics for any facility with low booster vaccine rates for staff and residents.

Short-term steps to improve nursing home staffing include introducing a Federal minimum staffing standard, increasing staff pay and benefits, providing opportunities for career advancement, and creating a better work environment.

In the longer run, the recent National Academies of Sciences, Engineering, and Medicine Committee on which I served concluded that the way in which the United States finances and regulates care in nursing home setting is ineffective, inefficient, fragmented, and unsustainable.

To create a more rational approach to financing nursing home care that would address these significant shortcomings, the National Academies report included a recommendation about moving toward a Federal long-term care benefit by studying how to design such a benefit and then implementing state demonstration programs to test the model prior to national implementation.

To ensure adequate investment in caring for long-stay nursing home residents, our study committee recommended the use of detailed and accurate financial information to ensure payments are adequate to cover comprehensive nursing home care.

We also recommended the designation of a specific share of Medicare and Medicaid payments go toward direct care services as opposed to noncare costs, such as lease payments. And we also recommended the increased use of value-based nursing home payment models to reward facilities for providing better quality.

In terms of regulatory reforms, the National Academies committee provided recommendations to ensure state survey agencies have adequate resources, and we made additional recommendations for the oversight of state survey performance.

In terms of increasing financial and ownership transparency, we recommended collecting, auditing and making detailed facility-level data on the finances, operation, and ownership of all nursing homes publicly available in real-time in a readily useable data base that allows for the assessment of quality by a common owner or management company.

In summary, the pandemic has indeed lifted the veil on nursing home care in America. We have an incredible opportunity right now to address problems that we have ignored for far too long.

I look forward to working with the members of this subcommittee on this effort. Thank you.

Mr. CLYBURN. Thank you very much, Dr. Grabowski.

We'll now hear from Ms. Ramos. Ms. Ramos, you are now recognized for five minutes.

Statement of Adelina Ramos, Certified Nursing Assistant, Greenville, Rhode Island

Ms. RAMOS. Thank you, Chairman Clyburn, Ranking Member Scalise, and the members of the committee for inviting me to speak today.

My name is Adelina Ramos. I'm a certified nurse assistant at a nursing home in Greenville, Rhode Island. I'm also a proud member of SEIU 1199 New England.

Like so many facilities across the country, we were not prepared for COVID. Our facility already had issues, and COVID made everything worse. When COVID first hit, three or four residents in my facility died each week. A CNA at my facility was one of the first nursing home workers to die of COVID in Rhode Island.

In May 2020, I got the news that I've been dreading for so long. I had COVID. I did everything I could not to catch the virus, but the conditions were so bad in my facility, it was impossible to avoid. It didn't have to be like this.

We needed personal protective equipment. We needed more training to keep ourselves and the residents safe. We need more staff. We pleaded with the management, but nothing changed.

Mother's Day 2020 really broke my heart. One of my residents was slipping away, and her children could not see her, and she wanted me to sit with her, but I couldn't because I was caring for 25 other residents. There was only a nurse, another CNA, and a housekeeper on that shift that day.

Most of those residents couldn't eat, drink, get out of bed, or go to the bathroom without help. They all required oxygen changed every 15 minutes. We regularly have to make impossible choices about which residents to help first. Do I go to the resident sit in a soiled bed, or do I go to a resident who fell and is asking for help? What if it happened—the fall happens while I'm toileting another resident.

Rushing can only cause more harm. Our residents' families trust us to care for their loved ones. I can't describe how painful it feels when we are forced to make those kinds of choices.

Today, I'm vaccinated. The vaccine and boosters have made a huge difference. We can care for our residents better, and they're not as scared of the virus; however, the crisis in our nursing homes is far from over. We continue to face a severe staffing shortage.

CNAs are burnt out mentally and physically. Our pay is so low that some of us have to work two or three jobs. Nursing home staff leave the work force for agencies because they pay higher. The residents want care from people they know and trust. They can get the right—I'm sorry.

They can't get that right now at my facility because the turnover in agency staff is in and out. We never know who will be there on a given day if there will be enough staff.

Residents are disappointed and frustrated. Some ask me, why can't we have more staff? And why can't they pay more? I also want to say that this isn't about CNAs. Every single nursing home job is essential—housekeepers, maintenance workers, nurses, dietary workers, aides, and activity workers, altogether, to give residents the best care possible and the best quality of life.

The majority of nursing home workers are women and people of color, and we are often called unskilled and uneducated. Our jobs are devalued. It's disgraceful. After 2–1/2 years of a daily pandemic, we're still treated this way.

We are fed up with the lack of respect nursing home owners and lawmakers show our work force. Change needs to happen now. One way we can do that is through unions. Our unions have secured additional sick leave and better health insurance.

We want guidelines to ensure that we have safe staffing levels more often. A union contract means management has to follow the rules; it means workers have a seat at the table, and it means we can fight for our residents to have better care, but not every nursing home has a union. The workers—and the residents are suffering.

I'm here today, again, representing the thousands of nursing home workers who are still fighting for what we deserve. Congress has the power to set standards in all nursing homes. You have the power to hold nursing home owners accountable and make sure that public dollars are used to improve care and care jobs, not increase profits.

We will need quality care—we all will need quality care at some point of our lives, and that can only happen with a skilled, strong work force that is respected, protected, paid, and staffed.

On behalf of all nursing home workers and our residents, please take action. Thank you.

Mr. CLYBURN. Thank you, Ms. Ramos.

We will now hear from Mr. Arbeeny. Mr. Arbeeny, you are recognized for five minutes.

Statement of Daniel Arbeeny, Son of Nursing Home Resident

Mr. ARBEENY. Thank you, Chairman Clyburn, Ranking Member Scalise, and members of the Select Subcommittee on the Coronavirus.

My name's Daniel Arbeeny, and I live on Amity Street in Brooklyn, New York. In one week in April, four family members died: — my father, my uncle, and my two close cousins of the virus. Three of them are in nursing homes.

It was—we reluctantly, at that time, joined the 100,000 other New Yorkers in what we call the New York COVID nursing home orphans. There were a lot of people.

Thank you for very much for hearing this, and appreciate the opportunity to speak about our personal family experience.

The GAO testimony last year pointed out that while nursing home residents are less than one percent of the population, at that time, they were nearly 30 percent of the COVID deaths. Thank you, Chairman, for pointing out its now 20 percent.

Those are the ones that we're supposed to love, honor, and protect, and we failed. We failed miserably. No family should go through this, and we all went through it. Many here lived it on the other side.

In New York state, the critical component was the March 25 directive compelling nursing homes to accept COVID-positive patients. My family has lived on the same block for five generations in Brooklyn. It's a wonderful heritage we were given, but more importantly, it's where my family has deep community roots.

My father was a vivacious 88-year-old man, still working and driving with a very sharp mind and a quick smile. He sat on the stoop of the house, always offering a smile, a helping hand, and a greeting to everybody regardless.

In short, my dad was in rehab to get strong right around the corner. From his window, he saw the rehab center. And was COVID-free up until the time of the Governor's March 25 order. It was the nursing home who actually came to us and told us about the order and how Cuomo and the state health commissioner refused to listen and just ignored their pleas. They even came up with options for the state, all ignored. Excellent options, mind you.

Despite 24-hour care, we brought our father home, gave him 24-hour care. A week later, he passed away.

We took a COVID test 12 hours before; he died 12 hours later. Twelve hours after that approximately, we got a COVID-positive test. Even nonmedical personnel, we knew it was senseless for state government to exercise the fullest of its powers to compel people with a highly contagious disease, a killing machine at the time, into nursing homes where the weakest and most vulnerable were confined.

What could they possibly be thinking? My brother and I, we talked about this my family, our friends, and those similarly situated like us.

Then the state legislature agreed with the Governor and gave blanket immunity to everybody. At that point, our family decided we were going to find the truth, and that's what we're going to focus on and meaningfully help those like us.

Thankfully, the media began to focus on the Cobble Hill Health Center, our local nursing home. Why? Because New York state had asked all the nursing homes what were the number of probable deaths from COVID. One out of over 600 nursing homes answered truthfully—five, 10, 15, and our nursing home said 55.

Well, the media, thankfully, descended on them. They were the canary in the coal mine. They truthfully answered. They truthfully answered, and the media were trying to skewer them. We spent hours speaking to every outlet you can imagine, AP, The Wall Street Journal, and CNN, to show them what was happening. And in the end, each one of them realized that had nothing to do with the nursing homes in New York, they were forced into this, and they had no idea about the March 25 order, the PPE shortages in the nursing homes that the state was ignoring.

On October 18, we held a mock funeral for our Governor's leadership and integrity, which focused on two simple things: An apology and the true death toll. That came about because he was writing a book on his leadership, and he had just published it. October, six months later?

Despite the fact that COVID being a virus, knows no political party; he blamed it on politics. Based on what we know today, every statistic New York state used was misleading. Rather than using facts to point us to the truth, the guardians of the public interest used their offices to point us away from the truth.

Finally, and thankfully, on January 2021, the state attorney general announced a bombshell report that the deaths were under-counted, and so were the readmissions. Speaking for myself and almost every other family member in this situation, we still have not accomplished our goal of learning the truth. And I'm here before you to hope that you can help us accomplish that.

No one in public or private sectors admitting the culpability for the death, distress, pain, and suffering that was caused and concealed; for this reason, we welcome the attention of this committee on the nursing home aspect of this American tragedy and urge further oversight and help.

Thank you.

Mr. CLYBURN. Thank you.

The chair now recognizes Dr. Travers for five minutes.

Statement of Jasmine Travers, Rn, Assistant Professor of Nursing, New York University, Rory Meyers College of Nursing

Ms. TRAVERS. Chairman Clyburn, Ranking Member Scalise, and members of the Select Subcommittee on the Coronavirus Crisis thank you for this invitation to speak today on the work force issues, equity, and disparities.

Several issues are inherent to the nursing home work force of many rooted and structural inequities. These inequities present as staffing shortages, inadequate pay and benefits, lack of advancement opportunities, and poor working conditions. Certified nursing assistants, and CNAs, bear the brunt.

When asked about the biggest challenge affecting nursing homes' day-to-day operations, administrators often mention insufficient staffing. Proposed minimum staffing hours had been defined, yet these levels are rarely met. Nursing homes, not meeting hours, have higher Medicaid census portions of Black residents, for-profit ownership, and located in severely deprived neighborhoods and rural settings.

Staff shortages have severe consequences for resident safety, quality of care, and job satisfaction. CNAs have reported being responsible for more than 20 to 30 residents simultaneously, creating heavy workloads and unhealthy working conditions.

Insufficient staffing can result from the inability for homes to recruit and retain staff and not scheduling enough staff. Such challenges center around stigma toward nursing homework, including the type of work, pay, and workload. Often staff receives less pay than peers working in other settings, such as hospitals or even other industries where the work is less demanding.

Last, funding the care of older adults has often been deprioritized in deference to childcare, critical care, and other specialties. Staffing interventions must address these issues.

Centers for Medicare and Medicaid services, hereafter referred to as CMS, intends to propose a minimum staffing standard next year. CMS is collecting information and opinions from staff residents and families. Vital for the success of the minimum staffing standard is supplying more funding.

As it stands, CMS is pushing states to use their Medicaid funding to improve nursing home funding and tie increases to accountability efforts, such as quality measures and higher staff wages; however, CMS must do more than encourage state action.

A strong commitment is needed to improve the working conditions and environment related to education and training, compensation and benefits, opportunities, empowerment, and treatment through mandates, incentives, and accountability efforts, along with temporary support, such as strike teams.

It is important to highlight this systemic inequities that have perpetuated disparities among nursing home residents. Homes with any Black residents experience significantly more COVID infections and deaths than homes with no Black residents.

Beyond the pandemic, when compared to the White counterparts, Black and Latino's residents are likelier to experience pressure ulcers and falls, and under treatment for pain, ordered antipsychotics and restraints, and less likely to receive preventive care.

Residents who identify as LGBTQ + or living with dementia often do not receive the required care because of limited staff knowledge and training on how to care for these groups, along with biases.

Failure to hire staff that is culturally congruent to residents results in inequitable care experiences when residents' cultural and linguistic preferences are unmet. To that end, all older adults deserve equitable care. Several recommendations in the National Academies reports speak to this.

First, identify care preferences and implement and monitor corresponding care plans. Second, ensure nursing homes are accountable for the total cost of care and poor care delivered through alternative payment models. Third, require staff participation in ongoing diversity, equity, and inclusion training.

Fourth, prioritize models that reduce disparities and strengthen connections to communities and broader healthcare systems. Last, develop a health equity strategy for nursing homes. This is important to know what additional work is needed and where.

Finally, I want to emphasize the importance of combining policies, data, and experience to truly appreciate the consequences of decreased oversight, support, and accountability.

During the pandemic, CMS waived inspection requirements outside of infection control. Thus citations for deficiencies such as odor and care planning were ignored. Visiting homes, my nose would sting from the pungent smells of urine and feces. Sheets were heavily soiled, and residents were severely unkempt. Pleas among residents for simple requests such as going outside just to feel the sun on their faces were constant yet unaddressed.

While such citations may seem unimportant, it leads to poor quality of care, such as falls, pressure ulcers, infections, depression, and avoidable hospitalizations and deaths. We must consider the lives that were lost for these reasons and approach such waivers more meaningfully in the future.

In conclusion, I urge the subcommittee to recognize that older adults do not want to stop living, although they might need help living. Only then we'll be able to start to make a meaningful change necessary to improve nursing home care for our staff, residents, and families.

And I just want to recognize Congresswoman Carolyn Maloney, who represents NYU. Thank you.

Mr. CLYBURN. Well, thank you very much, Dr. Travers. Each member will now have five minutes for questions.

The chair now recognizes himself for five minutes.

Thanks to the Biden/Harris administration's historic vaccination campaign, 87 percent of nursing home residents and 89 percent of staff have been vaccinated against the Coronavirus. These tremendous vaccination rates helped to curtail the devastation that we saw in nursing homes in 2020.

Ms. Ramos, you worked on the front lines of the coronavirus pandemic as a certified nursing assistant at a nursing home in Rhode Island. You've testified today that you had personal experiences that I would like for you to tell us what you think has been the impact of this Coronavirus on your life and the lives of the residents you cared for.

Ms. RAMOS. Thank you, Senator, for the question.

So on, 2020 was the worst day I've ever experienced in my whole life when we first got our residents that was sick with the virus. At that time, I was working on the dementia unit, which means that those residents couldn't tell us, like, their symptoms, how they were feeling.

We—our residents were falling, and then that's when we find out they were very weak and sick. And at that time that's when we kind of figured, like, they were getting sick and then they were trying to test them and to make sure they had the virus.

But for us, the staff, they weren't testing us at that time. So we had to go out on our own and, if we had the symptoms, to test ourselves. The facility wasn't doing that. And also, we didn't have enough PPE at the facility. We were told we had to use the same mask for several days and we have to reuse the gowns. And we were also told that what we were trained in infection or if you had any virus, we're supposed to change our PPE. And we were told that they didn't have enough.

So since the facility that I work at, we have a union. We had to call our union organizer and complain the situation that was going on at the facility, that some staff are having the symptoms and they were not testing them. And they would go out on their own and get tested, and that we didn't have enough PPE.

So our union had to bring us extra PPE, and also they had to call the state to come in and test us. That's how they send in the National Guard, and that's when I find out I was asymptomatic, and I find out that I was positive when the state came in.

Mr. CLYBURN. Can you tell me, did the vaccine, once the vaccine came, was there—what was the extent of the change?

Ms. RAMOS. So when we finally got the vaccine, I was actually one of the first ones in the group with my other colleagues that decided to go first because a lot of our colleagues weren't sure about the vaccine. They were kind of afraid of the symptoms, and they were afraid that they have to lose time from work.

And so our—, again, our unit had to make sure and, like, work with the management and told them that we're doing that for the best care of our residents and that we shouldn't be losing our pay if we get the symptoms.

So after we got the vaccine, our coworkers saw that, you know, we were doing better with the—symptoms weren't that bad. So— and also, our residents, some of our residents were very excited that we had the vaccine, and they were excited to get the vaccine.

So they went, and I got the vaccine. So after we got the vaccine, our residents and our staff members were very excited, and also our residents didn't die on the rate they were dying previously. So we probably had three—like one to two residents that died from COVID for the past year.

Before the vaccine, we lost like 20-plus residents at my facility.

Mr. CLYBURN. Well, thank you very much. I'm almost out of time.

I'll now yield to the ranking member.

Mr. SCALISE. I thank the Chairman again, and I appreciated all of the witnesses' testimoneys. As we covered in the beginning, we saw pretty early often in the pandemic as the CDC and CMS were putting out guidance and specifically for nursing homes, they were making it very clear that a nursing home shouldn't be taking patients if they didn't have a plan to keep COVID-positive patients separated. Yet, in fact, you saw New York, through Governor Cuomo, start issuing that order that, ultimately, then other states followed.

We saw New Jersey come right behind it, almost verbatim. And I'll read the New York guidance because it was then used by New Jersey, Michigan, California, and Pennsylvania went for it as well, and this is, quote, from the mandate from Governor Cuomo's health department: No resident shall be denied readmission or admission to the nursing home solely based on a confirmed or suspected diagnosis of COVID–19.

Nursing homes are prohibited from requiring a hospitalized resident who is determined medically stable to be tested for COVID– 19 prior to admission or readmission.

So there you have the Governor of New York saying, if you're a nursing home and there is a patient coming from a hospital, possibly COVID-positive, back into your nursing home, and you're not prepared to take care of that patient, you still have to take them going against guidance from CDC, and even further more egregious, you are banned from testing them for COVID.

And, of course, New York is the regulator of the nursing homes. And so Mr. Arbeeny, in your testimony, you pointed out that the nursing home saw this. They saw what was going on with COVID, the deaths that were happening, especially in the most vulnerable populations, and they knew this could be a huge problem, but their regulator's telling them, you got to do something that actually could undermine the health of your own residents, and they pleaded with the Governor not to do this.

If you can expand on that, what did you hear from the guy? Have you gotten a response from the Governor, because we surely haven't, and we've asked time and time again for the same numbers you're talking about. Still, if you could share—because that had to be a really frightening experience to be told by your regulator, you have to do something that you know could lead to the deaths of the very people you're there to protect?

Mr. ARBEENY. Thank you. It was—we knew at the time what was happening at the hospitals, which were struggling, too, with staffing, and we knew what was happening on our nursing home. And when they came to us and said, you can take better care of your father at home because you're engaged, you need to take him home, it was—it was like a hurricane.

I have no other way to describe how my family and I all got together and came up with a plan. The hospital had left some medical needs alone. They weren't doing anything unless it was life-threatening, so we had to get those taken care of.

It was—we were in a race for our lives, and we knew it, and we did everything in our power to get him home. And at the same time, we were going out, and—we made a donation. My family led a group donating to our local police station and twice to our local nursing home, thousands of pieces of PPE because we saw with our own eyes what was happening to our loved ones. We saw what was happening to our police. They had nothing.

So our city knew, our state knew what was happening, and they ignored it. Their focus was the hospital——

Mr. SCALISE. And did you get any reaction from Governor Cuomo or his office that they were,—I mean. Obviously, they're being told this could be deadly. Did they even care? Did they do anything differently?

Mr. ARBEENY. No, they did nothing differently. Our local elected officials sent emails, called. We had a fully functional ICU hospital one block from our house, one and a half blocks from the nursing home. They were, Please, use that building. It's the perfect building. Negative. Pressure rooms built specifically for this. Governor Cuomo would not use it.

Mr. SCALISE. Let me come back to that. I wanted to ask Dr. Grabowski because it seems like you've done some research. There's some pretty riveting numbers that you talked about, not only nursing home deaths, but especially 2,600 people who worked in nursing homes—it wasn't just the nursing home families, like you said, 100,000 families who were part of this orphan class now you're talking about, but those workers, were you aware of these mandates from the regulators, the states like New York who said you have to take them back and you can't test them for COVID?

Mr. GRABOWSKI. So we didn't study those directly in our research. We took a much more national focus, but certainly, I've since then heard a lot about the——

Mr. SCALISE. Does it sound like that followed CDC guidance to force them to do something that CDC was telling them not to do?

Mr. GRABOWSKI. Yes. So I didn't sort of get into that in my research at the time. We didn't focus a lot on kind of the New York and the timing of when CDC was releasing that guidance, so I wouldn't be the right person to comment on that.

Mr. SCALISE. Mr. Chairman, I'll yield back, but Mr. Arbeeny and every other family out there, we are not going to stop fighting to get those answers even if Governor Cuomo and others want to keep hiding the facts. We are going to dig until we get the answers to those questions.

I yield back.

Mr. CLYBURN. Thank you, Mr. Scalise.

The chair now recognizes Mrs. Maloney for five minutes.

Mrs. MALONEY. Thank you so much, Mr. Chairman, for calling this important hearing. Paid sick leave for nursing home workers allow staff to take care of themselves and their families and to keep residents safe, but shockingly, many nursing homes do not offer paid sick leave to workers at all.

This puts many staff in an impossible situation, particularly during outbreaks of infectious diseases like the Coronavirus.

Dr. Bonner, what impact does the lack of paid sick leave have on the health and well-being of both nursing home staff and the residents they care for? Ms. Bonner?

Ms. BONNER. Thank you for the question.

So I think it's significant that in nursing homes, not only things like lack of paid sick leave but other benefits may drive people to, you know, come to work even when they are not feeling well, even when they, you know, have sick children or sick older adults at home.

And so, you know, this has been identified in some of the studies that our colleagues have talked about today as, you know, one of the factors that may have led to spread of the coronavirus crisis more rapidly in, you know, organizations like nursing homes.

So there are over 500,000 CNAs who work in nursing homes and many other professionals, and, again, they felt a sense of duty to be there to take care of residents. And so the lack of paid sick leave—also, many of the people who are nursing-home workers are single parents. They've got children at home, and they've got bills to pay. And so, you know, without any paid sick leave, this was thought to be one of the challenges during the pandemic.

Mrs. MALONEY. Well, thank you.

Ms. Ramos, I understand that you have been caring for nursing-home residents throughout the pandemic and that the facility where you work does provide paid sick leave to you and your colleagues.

How has paid leave helped you and your coworkers do your jobs effectively during the pandemic? Ms. Ramos.

Ms. RAMOS. Thank you for your question.

So our facility does have sick leave. That's because it says in our union contract that we accumulate sick leave through the bargain that we did. And, also, we have a state sick leave that's, like, separate from our contract.

But at the beginning of the pandemic, we were also told that we had to use our sick time when we got COVID from work. So our union had to work with the management and negotiate with the management, saying to them they got sick from work, and they shouldn't be using their sick time to pay for them to be out because they got COVID from work.

So what ended up happening is that our union finally talked to the management, and they come up with, if we got COVID from work, we will go through workman's comp. And so that's how we got paid. And we were homesick, and then, whenever we got better, that's when we went back to work.

But for a lot of workers that are not—that have non-union facilities, I've heard from some of my friends that they had to go to work sick or else they would lose their jobs, they were told.

And some of them were actually sick at work until they couldn't be sick anymore, you know, they couldn't take it anymore, and they had to be out, but they were not getting paid. And I felt bad for one of my friends when she told me that, what was happening.

Thank you.

Mrs. MALONEY. Thank you.

Nursing-home workers, many of whom are women and people of color, also struggle with low pay and have high poverty rates. According to a 2022 report by PHI, a leading authority on the direct care work force, 12 percent of nursing assistants working in nursing homes live in a household below the Federal poverty line, and 34 percent rely on some form of public assistance.

This is not just an economic issue; it's a real-life consequence for nursing-home residents.

Dr. Grabowski, how does low pay for nursing-home workers create risk for nursing-home residents in addition to the staff?

Mr. GRABOWSKI. Thanks for that question.

Our nurse staff are heroes. We didn't treat them or pay them like heroes before the pandemic, and we certainly didn't treat them and pay them like heroes during the pandemic.

When we underpay staff, they leave these positions, there's huge staff turnover at these facilities, leading to gaps in care, discontinuities in care that leads to bad outcomes for our residents.

The best thing that we can do for our residents is support our staff. And that means paying them well, giving them strong benefits, like Ms. Ramos just described with paid sick leave, and really making it a job worth having.

Thanks.

Mrs. MALONEY. Thank you.

My time has expired, and I yield back.

Mr. CLYBURN. Thank you very much.

The chair now recognizes Mr. Jordan for five minutes.

Mr. JORDAN. Thank you, Mr. Chairman.

Dr. Grabowski, was it a bat, to a penguin, to a hippopotamus, to Joe Rogan, and Aaron Rodgers, or did COVID start in a lab? Dr. Fauci and Dr. Collins say it's the former; they said it was animal to human.

Some of the virologists who they've given our tax dollars to over the years have said the same—, although, initially, I think it's interesting to point out, before they had their conference call with Dr. Fauci and Dr. Collins on February 2, on January 31, 2020, Dr. Kristian Andersen, who's received a number of our tax dollars over the years, said "virus looks engineered," "virus not consistent with evolutionary theory." Dr. Garry said, "It's easy to do this in a lab." They, of course, changed their position after they had this famous conference call with Dr. Collins and Dr. Fauci.

I was just wondering what you think. Did it start in a lab, or was it from a bat, to a penguin, to a person?

Mr. GRABOWSKI. So, I'm a health economist. My research has been focused on nursing-home supporting staff, supporting residents——

Mr. JORDAN. You've got a degree—I saw your background. You've got a degree from Duke degree from Chicago. You're a professor of healthcare policy at Harvard.

Is it a good idea for the guys in charge of our government policy on this to mislead the American people?

Mr. GRABOWSKI. So, I don't have an opinion on where the virus started or——

Mr. JORDAN. Just last week, Dr. Redfield was interviewed, and Dr. Redfield said this: "Fauci knew he was misleading the Congress and the country."

Do you agree with Dr. Redfield, or do you think Dr. Fauci was telling us the truth?

Mr. GRABOWSKI. Once again, I don't have an opinion on this. This is sort of outside the scope of my——

Mr. JORDAN. When the government said the vaccinated couldn't get the virus, were they guessing or lying?

Mr. GRABOWSKI. Once again, this is sort of outside the scope of what I focus on. I'm really focused on the care of our nursing-home residents, in particular——

Mr. JORDAN. Yes, but you're a smart guy. You're a professor at the Harvard University School of Medicine.

Mr. GRABOWSKI. And I'm a smart guy that chooses to focus on nursing homes and really supporting those——

Mr. JORDAN. Well, how about this question? How about this—— Mr. GRABOWSKI [continuing]. And putting better nursing-home policies in place to really——

Mr. JORDAN. Well, can the vaccinated——

Mr. GRABOWSKI [continuing]. Provide better care for our residents and our staff.

Mr. JORDAN. Can the vaccinated get the virus?

Mr. GRABOWSKI. Sorry. Ask that again.

Mr. JORDAN. Can the vaccinated get the virus?

Mr. GRABOWSKI. Did individuals who were vaccinated get COVID?

Mr. JORDAN. Can they get it, yes.

Mr. GRABOWSKI. Sure.

Mr. JORDAN. Sure, they can. So when the government told us that they couldn't, were they guessing or lying?

Mr. GRABOWSKI. Once again, that's sort of outside the scope of what I——

Mr. JORDAN. How about this one? Is the pandemic over?

Mr. GRABOWSKI. Once again, that's not for someone in my position. I'm a health economist whose research focuses on nursing homes.

Mr. JORDAN. Yes, but you're in front of the—you're in front of the Select Committee on Coronavirus. I mean, we talked about the number today. I think you cited—Representative Scalise cited this as well. I think it was 172,000 individuals in nursing homes lost their lives. We're talking about healthcare policy.

One of the things it seems we should be getting to the bottom of is how did this thing start. You're a witness in front of the committee with this background—educated guy, professor of healthcare and policy at Harvard.

I'm just asking you something—the President of the United States seems to think the pandemic is over. I'm asking, do you think the pandemic's over?

Mr. GRABOWSKI. Once again, this is a hearing about nursing homes. I'm really focused on, how do we support our staff and how do we support our residents? And that's what my research——

Mr. JORDAN. Well, we might not have had the terrible things happen in nursing homes if the government would've been square with us from the get-go. That's one of the things I think is important for the country to understand. Maybe some of these terrible things don't happen.

In fact, we've had testimony in front of this committee that said if they would've focused on the idea that this came from a lab—and I asked Dr. Jarrar. I said, "Would that have changed how we dealt with the virus, and could that have saved lives," and he said, "Yes, it would've."

So that's why we're asking the question. That's why it's important to the American people. And, frankly, just on a fundamental level, it's important that the government not mislead its citizens, which it obviously seems they're doing.

So maybe I'll ask it this way now. If the pandemic's over—because the President said it just a couple days ago—and the government misled us on the origin of the virus—it seems pretty obvious they did. They definitely misled us on the statement that the vaccinated couldn't get it or transmit it—should people who lost their job be able to get it back?

Mr. GRABOWSKI. Once again, that's kind of outside the scope of kind of what I—what I research.

Mr. JORDAN. Recruitment levels for our military are off 40 percent. I just talked to colleagues on the House floor who say for the first time in their time as a Member of Congress where they didn't have as many apply to go into our academies, because of the vaccine—because of the vaccine mandate that's on.

I'm just asking the basic question, should people—healthcare policy. This seems to have a bearing on overall policy. Should people who lost their job be able to get it back, particularly in the United States military?

Mr. GRABOWSKI. So my research hasn't focused on, kind of, job loss in the military. That's really kind of outside the area that I study. I'm very focused on nursing homes, which is the focus of this hearing.

Mr. JORDAN. How about this one? Should Pfizer, J&J, Moderna have to pay the back-salary of people who lost their job, seeing how they've been misled on the effectiveness of this vaccine?

Mr. GRABOWSKI. Once again, that's not an issue that I've focused on in my research.

Mr. JORDAN. Mr. Chairman, I yield back.

Mr. CLYBURN. I thank the gentleman for yielding back. The chair now recognizes Mr. Foster for five minutes.

Mr. FOSTER. Yes, thank you, Mr. Chair.

And I guess I'd like to start by apologizing on behalf of the U.S. Congress, you know, and to express my admiration for your not getting lured into trying to talk about things where you don't have the training or the knowledge about. As you can see, the U.S. Congress is not constrained in that way, for talking about things we know nothing about.

Mr. JORDAN. Do you think knowing where this thing started is important?

Mr. FOSTER. Reclaiming my time, I would like to actually at this point ask you——

Mr. JORDAN. Well, I mean, this is a fundamental question. This is the Select Committee on the Coronavirus.

Mr. CLYBURN. Mr. Jordan——

Mr. JORDAN. The origin of the virus is an important——

Mr. FOSTER. Reclaiming my time——

Mr. JORDAN [continuing]. Question, Mr. Chairman.

Mr. CLYBURN. Mr. Jordan, I think you know that I'm not going to tolerate that.

Mr. JORDAN. Well——

Mr. CLYBURN. No one has disrupted you.

Mr. JORDAN. No, but he commented——

Mr. CLYBURN. No——

Mr. JORDAN [continuing]. About my questioning, and I'm asking a fundamental question.

Mr. FOSTER. I commented on my time. And I will continue to use my time——

Mr. JORDAN. About my questions.

Mr. FOSTER. Correct. And that's——

Mr. JORDAN. You can ask whatever questions——

Mr. CLYBURN. No——

Mr. JORDAN [continuing]. You want. You don't have to comment about mine. And if you comment about mine, I want to raise the fundamental question, why won't this committee look into how this thing started?

Mr. CLYBURN. I answered your question, and you aren't going to ask a question again now. I'm going to ask you very politely to——

Mr. JORDAN. Obviously——

Mr. CLYBURN [continuing]. Recognize and respect——

Mr. JORDAN. Mr. Chairman——

Mr. CLYBURN [continuing]. The gentleman's time.

Mr. JORDAN [continuing]. Obviously, the Democrats don't care about finding out how this virus that disrupted so many lives, including Mr. Arbeeny's family—they don't care about finding how this thing started.

Mr. CLYBURN. My family has been——

Mr. JORDAN. I do, and the folks I represent do.

Mr. CLYBURN. Your family has been impacted by this, and so has mine. So let's stay away from that.

Mr. JORDAN. So I'd think you would like to know how—I think it makes sense for you——

Mr. CLYBURN. And I've got——

Mr. JORDAN [continuing]. To question how this thing started.

Mr. CLYBURN [continuing]. Enough sense to know that we are going to do this in regular order. And the order here today is to talk about nursing homes. We are not going to get into that.

Mr. JORDAN. You've yet to get into it in two years that we've had——

Mr. CLYBURN. Mr. Foster?

Mr. FOSTER. Yes. Thank you, Mr. Chair.

And I also—I, too, lost my favorite aunt and my favorite uncle in a nursing home in the situation. And I just want to say that the vast majority of people working in the nursing-home industry were trying to do the right thing with imperfect information.

You know, it was months before we knew that this was primarily aerosol and that all of the business of sterilizing your food and superwashing your hands was largely irrelevant, and what was important is not to exhale in the presence of people who are vulnerable. OK? And it took us a while to understand just how simple that was.

Also, I'm a little bit concerned that we're trying to focus too much on what happened in certain—there were problems all over the country. And I'd like to at this point ask unanimous consent to put into the record a list prepared by staff of other states that had very significant problems—you know, Georgia, you name it—large— Connecticut, Maryland—just all over the country.

Mr. CLYBURN. Without objection.

Mr. FOSTER. And my aunt and uncle passed away in Pennsylvania, and I thought that staff there were doing the best they could under terrible circumstances.

And the way patients passed away, you know, being unable to talk to their loved ones, was tragic and, unfortunately, necessary, given what we knew about the virus then and what we know now, actually.

And there's a large number of lessons to be learned. One of them, too, is, as has been mentioned, the fact that we have been under-investing in the end-of-life care in this country for a long time. There is enough money in our country to solve this problem. It is not like we're asking for something that's unachievable.

You know, since the start of the Obama recovery, the net worth of Americans has increased from $60 trillion to nearly $150 trillion. All right? That's a lot of money. But unfortunately, not much of that increase in wealth has ended up in those in the middle class who fall out of the middle class at the end of life. Because that is who ends up in nursing homes.

This is not something just—you know, nursing homes are not just for minorities. And there's a sort of narrative about "this is what nursing homes are about," and it's not. It is ordinary, middle-class people who simply run out of resources at the end of their life.

And we have enough money to fix this in this country, and it is to our shame that we don't.

It was one of the first things I did when I was elected, geez, about 12 years ago, I guess. I asked: What, in Illinois, does your life look like when you run out of assets at the end of your life?

And there's a certain amount of money that we have. It's made much worse in Illinois, in fact, because Illinois, like New York, like California, and a number of other states, writes an enormous check to the Sunbelt and to the low-population western states. If we simply had—because we pay a lot more in Federal taxes than we get back in Federal spending.

That alone, fixing that, would provide a much better level of healthcare generally and particularly end-of-life care in states like New York and Illinois, and California, the large-population states who are routinely rooked by formula-driven spending from the U.S. Senate.

That's not the subject of this hearing, but it's really important when you talk about what's going on in individual states is the balance of payments between the states.

So I'd like to just talk a little bit about the labor force shortage here. You know, there's an obvious solution to this. It is called immigration reform. And there are hordes of very competent, well-trained nurses around the world. And they traditionally have entered the U.S. work force. They enter the U.S. and then start qualifying to get nursing credentials. They work as ordinary nursing assistants in eldercare homes. I visited one just a few weeks ago here.

And this is an obvious solution. And is there any reason that you've come to understand about why we can't fix this? Because it's all Americans who suffer from the lack of assistance.

Yes, Dr. Grabowski, any——

Mr. GRABOWSKI. Yes, sure.

So a large share of our labor force in nursing homes are currently immigrants. And I think as you're suggesting, Congressman, we could expand that, and we need to expand that going forward, especially with the aging baby-boom generation.

We're doing a study right now, and it fits exactly with what you're asking. It turns out areas with greater immigration see an increase in the work force in nursing homes, and guess what: It leads to better quality.

And so that link is absolutely there. We need to encourage strong pathways to get more immigrants in because that's going to be a big part of the puzzle. It's not the only piece, but it's going to be a big part of it going forward. We cannot do this on just using domestic workers alone. We're going to need strong immigration going forward.

Mr. FOSTER. OK. Thank you.

My time is up, and I yield back.

Mr. CLYBURN. If you have another question, I'm going to allow it because I think we took a minute and a half of your time listening to some foolishness. So I will allow you——

Mr. FOSTER. Yes, OK.

I guess, what we talked about,—you know, I'm a scientist, so I look for technological solutions that will make things better. And one of the things that strikes me is that there are a,—you know, diabetes is one-third of our healthcare costs. And there are treatments that are now looking like they're home runs in treating obesity and diabetes. You see them on TV, which—I won't quote the trade names, but you see them all the time.

And so the question that I have is, we've learned in COVID there are huge advantages in giving away certain things, like vaccines and testing, for free and that they net out as a huge savings in quality of life as well as taxpayer savings.

And I was wondering if there are ongoing ways—what is the framework for studying that and understanding if we can save the taxpayer money by distributing these diabetes cures, you know, for free to everyone?

Sure, yes. That sounds like healthcare economics.

Mr. GRABOWSKI. All right. I'll take that one.

Absolutely, there's a whole area of economics called value-based insurance design, where you lower the cost-sharing, maybe even make it zero, as you suggested, for high-value drugs and interventions. This might be an example of one such drug.

In order to study the savings with nursing homes, you'd really want to think about, what are the changes in functioning that this kind of drug might have for nursing-home residents?

Remember, for most nursing-home residents, Medicare is going to be paying for their healthcare, so a lot of the savings would be on the Medicare side, presumably, in terms of their healthcare spending. But are there savings on the nursing-home side, in terms of, you know, their functioning gets better, as you mention, maybe obesity is lower?

There are all sorts of ways that they may potentially end up costing Medicaid and Medicare less in the nursing home, and that's where we'd want to focus on and see if there's any potential offset there.

Mr. FOSTER. Thank you. And we'll be following up with you on that.

Mr. GRABOWSKI. All right. Thank you.

Mr. CLYBURN. Thank you very much.

The chair now recognizes Dr. Green for five minutes.

Mr. GREEN. Thank you, Mr. Chairman.

Mr. Grabowski, I'm going to be submitting a question in writing to you.

Mr. GREEN. But, Mr. Chairman, I'm yielding my time to the gentlelady from New York, Ms. Stefanik.

Ms. STEFANIK. Thank you, Dr. Green.

Mr. Arbeeny, thank you so much for being here today as an advocate on behalf of so many New York families, the 100,000 New York COVID orphans, essentially, for the over 10,000 lost loved ones in nursing homes.

I want to start off on March 25, when Governor Cuomo issued that fatal directive, forcing nursing homes to accept COVID-positive patients. Did you consider that a death sentence for the most vulnerable in New York's nursing homes?

Mr. ARBEENY. We absolutely did. And not just myself, not just my siblings, everybody we spoke to, whether they were in nursing homes, whether they were in hospitals, we all did. And we were all dumbfounded because we all knew the USS Comfort was sailing in. I went with my son and my wife to see it sail in.

Unfortunately, five days later, New York City had 3,000-plus beds that were never used——

Ms. STEFANIK. That's correct.

Mr. ARBEENY [continuing]. In the Javits Center and the USS Comfort. And the reason they weren't used was our state layered on top of the Federal admission policies their own admission policies, which I have access to, and so it was never used.

Ms. STEFANIK. It was a disaster. And I've spoken with constituents in my district, in New York 21, who lost their loved ones in nursing homes in the north country and upstate New York.

But I want to point out everyone knew Governor Cuomo and Lieutenant Governor Hochul's directive was not according to CMS guidance.

Look at this. Secretary of HHS: "There is no CDC guideline saying you should be taking positive COVID patients and putting them back in the community in nursing homes."

Former CMS Administrator Seema Verma: "Under no circumstances should a hospital discharge a patient to a nursing home that is not prepared to take care of those patient needs." And then, when asked directly, would New York state's guidance have violated CMS guidance, the answer was yes.

This was a death sentence.

And isn't it true that, only four days after issuing that directive, during Andrew Cuomo's press conference, he himself said that, quote, "Coronavirus and a nursing home is a toxic mix" and can be like, quote, "fire through dry grass?" Isn't it true that he said that?

Mr. ARBEENY. He said that multiple times. And I can actually get out the dates he said that. It was horrific for anybody that was living through that. Yes.

Ms. STEFANIK. So Governor Cuomo knew, and they worked overtime to cover this up. As families came forward,— they certainly came and tried to reach the Governor, tried to share their views, as well as the nursing-home workers—what was the Governor focused on? He was focused on winning his Emmy, which has since been taken away from him, and he was focused on cooking the books, withholding the numbers, so he could get his $5.2 million book contract, which was unethical.

I will always fight for transparency and answers.

My question is: Since Governor Cuomo has been forced to resign, Kathy Hochul, who was the sitting Lieutenant Governor, she promised to fight for transparency. She lied when she said that.

Can you talk about your family's experience, working with other advocates, your reaching out to Kathy Hochul, and what she has failed to do?

Mr. ARBEENY. My brother printed this out. This is my father's death certificate. And we've shown this to our attorney general, our comptroller, and we gave a copy to our current Governor. And she said she was mortified that she couldn't—, and nobody could tell us if my father's death counted, and that she wanted to get a true death count, that we shouldn't 50 years from now be trying to figure out what happened.

Unfortunately, nothing has happened. And as best we've been told through somebody else, they won't be looking back; they only want to look forward.

Ms. STEFANIK. She lied. And she continues to delay any investigation. She has refused to respond to congressional outreach from myself, Ranking Member Scalise, and Ranking Member Jamie Comer.

Isn't it true that the state senate, which is held by Democrats, they've refused to do a fulsome investigation into this?

Mr. ARBEENY. Yes. They have not done an investigation with subpoena power, and they've whitewashed it.

And we know this very clearly because of the attorney general, in January 2021, and our state comptroller came out with—sorry, 2022—and our state comptroller came out with their findings. And I could read to you those findings. I have the quotes. But at the very highest levels in our state government, we were lied to for their narrative.

Ms. STEFANIK. Help is on the way. The subpoenas are coming. House Republicans are committed to standing up and demanding answers and justice for those families that our colleagues across the aisle in New York state and here have failed to do.

The subpoenas are coming. Help is on the way.

I yield back.

Mr. CLYBURN. I thank the gentlelady for yielding back.

The chair now recognizes Mr. Raskin for five minutes.

Mr. RASKIN. Mr. Chairman, thank you very much.

This morning, this subcommittee released reports exposing the truly horrifying conditions in nursing homes across the country in the early months of the pandemic.

And I can remember like it was yesterday how the Trump administration abandoned nursing-home workers and other essential workers as they pleaded for the Federal Government to help them get critical supplies necessary to protect themselves on the job and curb the spread of the virus.

But, instead of mobilizing a serious Federal response, President Trump contemptuously stated that his administration was, quote, "not a shipping clerk," and he told the states to go and find their own supplies.

Today, I'm actually reading about a new book that's been published quoting Melania Trump in a phone call with former New Jersey Governor Christie, in which she discussed seeking help convincing her husband to take the pandemic more seriously.

"'You're blowing this,' she recalled telling her husband," the authors write. "'This is serious. It's going to be really bad. And you need to take it more seriously than you're taking it.' He just dismissed her. 'You worry too much,' she remembered him saying. 'Forget it.'"

The new documents demonstrate just how severely nursing-home facilities were affected by PPE shortages under the dereliction of duty of the administration.

So, long before Donald Trump did nothing to rescue his own Vice President, Mike Pence, as he was being hounded and chased out of the Capitol by Trump's mob, he was doing nothing to rescue tens of millions of Americans from the nightmare of COVID–19.

Some employees were reportedly told to, quote, "share PPE" with other employees. Some were only given one protective face mask to wear for an entire week and were instructed to use makeshift isolation gowns out of plastic or paper bags that were, quote, ''stapled and taped together.''

Ms. Ramos, as someone who worked in a nursing home during those early months of the pandemic, how did these systemic PPE shortages affect you and the lives and work of your colleagues?

Ms. RAMOS. Thank you for your question, Senator.

So, during that time, we didn't have enough PPE, like I said. We were struggling to get PPE. Like, we didn't have—they told us to use the same mask over and over again, and they told us to reuse the gowns.

So we also had—when our staff members were getting sick, we didn't have enough staff to work either. So we were short-staffed at that time also.

And during that time, we called our organizer and let them know what was going on in our facilities. And our organizer had to come for our rescue and bring us the PPE and also tell them that they need to do something about the staffing or the management has to come in and help out because we didn't have enough staffing.

Like, on Mother's Day, I remember clear that day, we had 26 residents that were very sick. And one of my residents, she asked me if I could stay by her bedside and hold her hand because her children were outside the window, visiting her. And it broke my heart because we didn't have enough staff on. So there were only 2 CNAs working that day and a nurse working that day, for 26 residents. And so it broke my heart, because I told her I couldn't sit with her because I have other 25 residents that I had to care for.

But we called the management, and the answer was we had enough staff on. And the PPE, our organizer, had to drop off some PPE.

But, also, the short-staffing, it didn't start with the pandemic. It also start before the pandemic. We had a big shortage of staff. So the pandemic made things worse for us in the nursing homes.

Mr. RASKIN. Well, thank you very much for your service and also for your testimony.

The previous administration's refusal or complete inability to do their job allowed one of the worst pandemics in history to run practically unchecked here in the United States.

Dr. Grabowski, how did the Trump administration's failure to provide nursing homes with PPE and other essential health supplies affect their ability to care for residents in the first months of the pandemic?

Mr. GRABOWSKI. Yes. Thanks for that question.

As Chairman Clyburn mentioned during my introduction, I served on the Trump administration's CMS Coronavirus Commission back in 2020. And we were asked to take stock of what had happened up until that point and offer a series of recommendations to really provide nursing homes with a roadmap out of the kind of crisis that they were in at the time.

And our recommendations included personal protective equipment, testing, support for staff like Ms. Ramos, better ventilation, and on and on and on—better data. All these issues have come up. Mr. Arbeeny talked about PPE and more transparency of data. You know, we had a really strong list of recommendations.

Those recommendations were not incorporated. The administration said, "Thank you," but didn't put them into practice. And I think that cost us a lot of lives at the time.

Congressman, if we had went ahead and really provided PPE to facilities, rapid testing, support for our staff, and on and on and on down the list, I think that death total I cited earlier would be a lot lower today.

Mr. RASKIN. Thank you for your testimony.

I yield back, Mr. Chairman.

Mr. CLYBURN. I thank the gentleman for yielding back.

The chair now recognizes Ms. Malliotakis for five minutes.

Ms. MALLIOTAKIS. Thank you, Mr. Chairman.

And thank you to our witnesses for being here today. As a New Yorker, I'm especially happy to welcome Mr. Arbeeny here to tell his story.

I think we could learn a lot from you and expose the decisions that were made by the Cuomo-Hochul administration that ultimately led to over 17,000 of our seniors dying and, unfortunately, your father. And my condolences for that.

I just want to talk about the timeline. Because on March 13, 2020, CDC and CMS released guidance stressing that a COVID– 19-positive nursing-home resident must be quarantined and properly treated. The guidance directly forbids nursing homes from accepting patients they were unable to properly treat.

Then, on March 15, in a phone call between Jared Kushner and Governor Cuomo, Cuomo allegedly said, "For nursing homes, this could be like fire through dry grass." He admitted that.

And March 19, the Society for Post-Acute and Long-Term Care Medicine warned, "Admitting patients with suspected or documented COVID–19 infection represents a clear and present danger to all the residents of a nursing home."

So it was very clear, very well known to everyone, that the elderly were the most vulnerable to COVID and that putting positive patients in the nursing home just lacked common sense.

On March 24, it was during his daily press briefing—, and it was very famous this video clip, where he said, "My mother is not expendable, and your mother is not expendable." And yet the very next day is when he put out that directive, that lethal directive, that mandated nursing homes, regardless of their ability to provide care, to accept the COVID–19-positive patients discharged from hospitals. And that directive prohibited the nursing homes from even testing the patients prior to admittance.

And, to boot, the state didn't even provide the PPE to help the nursing homes. And, like you said, you were delivering PPE. So was I, going to the nursing homes to try to help them, because they were forced to do this without any help from the Cuomo administration.

And it was directly against the CDC and CMS guidance and common sense.

Now, this is an interesting thing. Even after the Governor set up and the President sent in the USS Comfort ship, the DOD set up the Javits Center, on Staten Island, we had the South Beach Psych Center, even after there were alternatives that were not full, right, hardly used really, the Governor kept this mandate and kept requiring that nursing homes take that.

Why do you think that is?

Yes, Mr.—I would love—why do you think, even after——

Mr. ARBEENY. Yes.

Ms. MALLIOTAKIS [continuing]. There were alternatives, that he continued to put those positive patients in nursing homes?

Mr. ARBEENY. It's dumbfounding to me. And the way I'd like to answer it is: I could guess, but what I'd like to do is point out some facts.

On March 19, he started working with book publishers on his book our former Governor. And four months later, he all of a suden has a book and a book deal, and he's lying about all the numbers.

He called the President at the time, President Trump, and asked for help. President Trump set up, in less than 10 days, 3,000—almost 3,000 beds—no, 2,000 beds at the Javits Center. They mobilized. And five days after March 25th-ish, they all are open.

We did a FOIA request and found out, on April 7, the vice admiral in charge of those facilities was emailing the executive chamber and saying, "We have nobody here. Please send us,"—and you see the chain of emails. They're getting the runaround.

I can only guess that our Governor—, who then purposely made sure no one could use the Javits Center or the USS Comfort, because he layered admission policies on top of that,— didn't want to do it because it might make the President look good or it might help New Yorkers.

I can't understand how you could not do it.

Ms. MALLIOTAKIS. No.

I think we should also look into whether nursing homes got higher reimbursements than if he had put—would the state have gotten more money putting people in nursing homes or hospitals versus the alternative sites. That's something that should be looked at.

But one question. You mentioned your father was in the nursing home from—when? When did he start being in the nursing home?

Mr. ARBEENY. I don't remember the exact date for——

Ms. MALLIOTAKIS. Uh-huh.

Mr. ARBEENY [continuing]. The last one, but I think it was around March 25, plus or minus a couple——

Ms. MALLIOTAKIS. March 25. So it was before the directive.

Mr. ARBEENY. Yes, it was—I think it was—, sorry. It was a week before.

Ms. MALLIOTAKIS. So he was in that nursing home a week prior to the directive. The directive happens. And you're saying in April is when your father was positive and passed away. And, at that time, there were these alternatives set up.

Mr. ARBEENY. Correct.

Ms. MALLIOTAKIS. So you believe if Cuomo decided to put these individuals in the alternatives instead of the nursing home, your father could still be alive today?

Mr. ARBEENY. So the answer is, absolutely. I'm sure the staff brought the virus in. No one could say no to that. But putting 9,000 COVID-positive patients into the nursing homes is nothing short of a death sentence for my dad and the other tens of thousands of—15,000 people.

Ms. MALLIOTAKIS. Yes.

Well, again, my condolences. And I've run out of time, but thank you for being here.

Mr. ARBEENY. Thank you. Sorry for going over.

Mr. CLYBURN. I thank the gentlelady for yielding back.

The chair now recognizes Dr. Miller-Meeks for five minutes.

Mrs. Miller-Meeks. Thank you, Mr. Chair.

And I want to thank all of our witnesses for being here today. And let me also say to all of those who lost loved ones during the COVID–19 pandemic, as a physician and a former public health director, we know that infectious diseases are something that we have largely tried to help, to assist with, and COVID–19 is one of those where we still don't even know the origins of COVID–19 and are still uncertain about transmission status with vaccination, but we know people with vaccines and boosters can still transmit the virus. So we still have some to learn.

But one of the things I can say that we do know from the infectious disease and medical standpoint is that when you mix sick people with an infectious disease with well people that, you're likely to get transmission.

And as we've heard from my colleagues today, it's clear that the Governors in New York, New Jersey, and Michigan violated clear guidance and infectious-disease protocols by issuing must-admit orders, which sadly led to thousands of unnecessary elder deaths.

We already knew from the evidence we had from China that there was transmission in elderly people, that children rarely got ill. There was a question whether children would transmit the virus because they have a much better immune system. We knew that this group was the most susceptible group. And we already knew that there was guidance from CMS and from CDC in regards to admission status.

Let me also say that the actions of these Governors went against CMS and CDC guidance when they forced COVID–19-positive residents back into nursing homes, forced them to be accepted, and declined—and sometimes actually tried to get them not to test the COVID–19 status.

While the Trump administration was issuing guidance to attempt to protect this already-vulnerable population, these Governors showed carelessness and acted directly against the science.

This is not political. It's scientific. For those of you who have children and have gone into a pediatrician's office, most pediatricians' offices will segregate out the well children from the sick children. And, in fact, we did that with pathways into hospitals throughout the COVID–19 pandemic.

Long-term-care facilities have always been more vulnerable to infection, and infectious-disease outbreaks, for a plethora of reasons, but especially because they're primarily occupied by elder people who have an already-suppressed immune system. And this has remained true with COVID–19. However, carelessness and a lack of following the science led to worse outcomes than what was necessary.

And I would say any public health director, state public health director—and I was one in Iowa,— would have known that putting COVID–19-positive patients or patients who had not fully recovered from a COVID–19 diagnosis and admission to a hospital would put others at risk.

When the population of caregivers is primarily younger, who may not get ill, it's possible they could bring in COVID–19 coming into a facility, but more likely introduced from ill patients who had poor immune systems and were more likely to transmit.

So I believe that, as we look back and conduct oversight of the COVID–19 pandemic, we should look at the importance of ensuring long-term-care facilities remain a priority when it comes to allocation of resources such as PPE and vaccines for situations such as when the pandemic arises in the future.

And, Mr. Arbeeny, I think you've spoken to this, but could you speak to the risk this presents to residents of nursing homes.

And can anyone provide a good explanation for the inconsistencies in how we did in hospitals, acute-care hospitals, in segregating patients, and then what was allowed to be admitted and mandated in New York, New Jersey, and in Michigan?

Mr. ARBEENY. It felt to me, in my experience being in the hospital system and in the nursing-home system, that—or, not "it felt to me,"—all the focus in the media and everything our former Governor was saying was on the hospitals, not on the nursing homes. It felt like nursing homes were the orphaned stepchild. I can't put it any other way. And yet the nursing homes are where our most loved people are—our parents, our grandparents.

It was just—nobody with common sense would've ever done anything like that. And, what, 50 states—, 45 states didn't do that. The five that did, from what I remember—and I don't remember the numbers—, the outcomes were just so much higher.

Mrs. Miller-Meeks. And at a time when we prevented family members from being with those individuals.

Thank you so much for your testimony.

Mr. Chair, I yield back.

Mr. CLYBURN. I thank the gentlelady for yielding back.

Before we close, I ask unanimous consent to enter into the record 27 letters the committee has received from individuals and organizations about this crucial issue.

Without objection, so ordered.

Mr. CLYBURN. In closing, I want to thank all of today's witnesses for their testimony. We appreciate your insight and expertise as we seek to understand the challenges that America's nursing homes faced during the coronavirus crisis so we can learn from the past and prepare for the future.

I also wish to apologize for the outburst we heard here today. When I was leaving home, going away to college, back in 1957, my dad shared with me a little anecdote, and he concluded with this thought: "Now, son," he said to me, "the first sign of a good education is good manners."

I've held to that. And it seems to me that a lot of people who went off to college did not get a good education. And so I apologize for what you were subjected to here today.

And I'm grateful that the Biden administration is focused on improving nursing homes in America so the Coronavirus and other infectious diseases no longer pose a dangerous threat to residents and staff.

Vaccinations, including being up to date on boosters, remain our most important tool in preventing severe outcomes from the Coronavirus. Nowhere has the life-saving impact of coronavirus vaccines been more apparent than in our Nation's nursing homes. And I am very pleased to hear your testimony here today, Ms.

Ramos, on that subject.

I urge all Americans to get vaccinated and to go out and get the updated bivalent booster as soon as they are eligible.

With that—and, without objection, all members will have five legislative days within which to submit additional written questions for the witnesses to the chair, which will be forwarded to the witnesses for their response.

Chapter 2

COVID-19 in Nursing Homes: Most Homes Had Multiple Outbreaks and Weeks of Sustained Transmission from May 2020 through January 2021*

United States Government Accountability Office

Abbreviations

CDC	Centers for Disease Control and Prevention
CMS	Centers for Medicare & Medicaid Services
COVID-19	Coronavirus Disease 2019
HHS	Department of Health and Human Services

Why GAO Did This Study

The COVID-19 pandemic has had a disproportionate impact on the 1.4 million elderly or disabled residents in the nation's more than 15,000 Medicare- and Medicaid-certified nursing homes. The Centers for Medicare & Medicaid Services (CMS) is responsible for ensuring that nursing homes nationwide meet federal quality standards.

The CARES Act includes a provision directing GAO to monitor the federal pandemic response. GAO was also asked to review CMS oversight of

* This is an edited, reformatted and augmented version of the United States Government Accountability Office Report to Congressional Addressees, Publication No. GAO-21-367, dated May 2021.

In: COVID-19 in Nursing Homes
Editor: Fred C. Wallace
ISBN: 979-8-88697-673-1

nursing homes in light of the pandemic. This report describes the frequency and duration of COVID-19 outbreaks in nursing homes. Future GAO reports will further examine nursing homes' experiences with COVID-19 outbreaks.

To conduct this work, GAO analyzed CDC data on COVID-19 reported by nursing homes each week of the review period from May 2020 through January 2021, the most recent data available at the time GAO conducted its review. Using CDC's definition of an outbreak, GAO determined the number and duration of outbreaks each nursing home experienced during the review period. GAO included data from the 13,380 Medicare- and Medicaid-certified homes (88 percent of Medicare- and Medicaid-certified homes) that passed CDC and CMS quality checks each week of the review period—the most reliable data for calculating the number and duration of outbreaks. GAO also categorized the nursing homes into two groups based on the duration of their longest outbreak: 1) those nursing homes with outbreaks lasting less than 5 weeks and 2) those nursing homes with outbreaks lasting at least 5 weeks.

What GAO Found

GAO analysis of data from the Centers for Disease Control and Prevention (CDC) shows that, from May 2020 through January 2021, nursing homes commonly experienced multiple COVID-19 outbreaks. According to CDC, an outbreak starts the week a nursing home reports a new resident or staff COVID-19 case and ends when there are 2 weeks with no new cases. GAO found that nursing homes had an average of about three outbreaks during the review period, with most of the nursing homes (94 percent, or 12,555 of the 13,380 nursing homes) experiencing more than one COVID-19 outbreak.

For each nursing home's longest- lasting COVID-19 outbreak, GAO found that about 85 percent (11,311 nursing homes) had outbreaks lasting 5 or more weeks. Conversely, for about 15 percent of nursing homes (2,005 homes), the longest outbreak was shorter in duration, lasting between 1 and 4 weeks, with 267 of those homes able to control their outbreaks after the initial week.

- The average number of COVID-19 cases per outbreak for nursing homes with a long-duration outbreak was 56, while the average for nursing homes with a short-duration outbreak was 13.

DURATION OF LONGEST COVID-19 OUTBREAK IN 13,316 NURSING HOMES

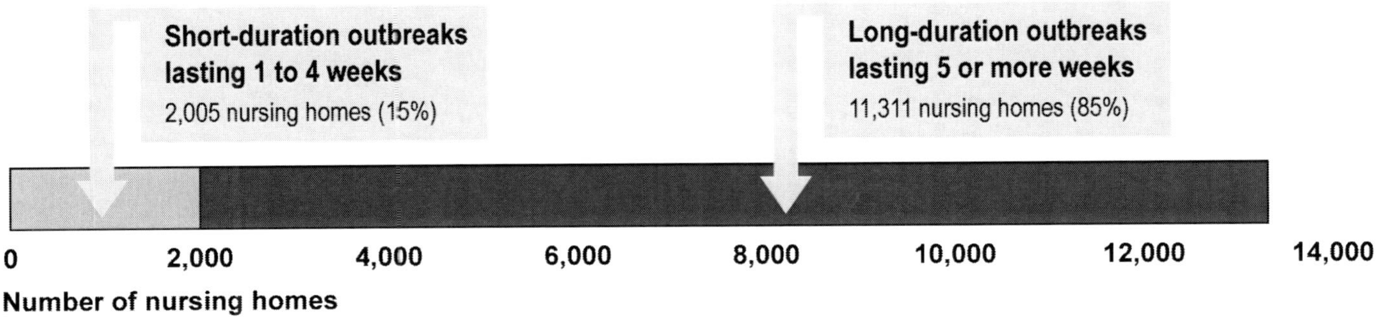

Source: GAO analysis of Centers for Disease Control and Prevention data.| GAO-21-367.

Note: Of 13,380 nursing homes reviewed, 13,316 nursing homes had COVID-19 outbreaks and 64 nursing homes did not. Data are from the weeks ending May 31, 2020, through January 31, 2021.

For both long- and short-duration outbreaks, over half of the nursing homes (66 percent, or 8,720 homes) reported that these outbreaks began with a staff member who tested positive the first week.

Letter

May 19, 2021

Congressional Addressees

The Coronavirus Disease 2019 (COVID-19) pandemic has had a disproportionate impact on the 1.4 million elderly or disabled residents in the nation's more than 15,000 Medicare - and Medicaid-certified nursing homes, who are often in frail health and living in close proximity to one another. One of the first major COVID-19 outbreaks was reported in a Washington State nursing home in February 2020, where there were reports that infection transmission continued among residents, staff, and visitors for several weeks before the outbreak was contained. One year later, the COVID-19 pandemic had reached nearly all Medicare- and Medicaid-certified nursing homes, according to data from the Centers for Disease Control and Prevention (CDC). While the introduction of vaccines and the sharp decline in nursing home cases and deaths since their peaks in December 2020 may indicate that nursing homes are seeing a reprieve, little is still known about the frequency and duration of COVID-19 outbreaks in nursing homes at critical points during the pandemic.

The CARES Act includes a provision directing us to monitor the federal response to the COVID-19 pandemic.[1] In response to the CARES Act, we have examined the response to COVID-19 in nursing homes in five reports since June 2020.[2] Also, you asked us to examine the Centers for Medicare & Medicaid Services' (CMS) oversight of infection prevention and control protocols and the adequacy of emergency preparedness standards for

[1] Pub. L. No. 116-136, § 19010(b), 134 Stat. 281, 579 (2020).

[2] We regularly issue government-wide reports on the federal response to COVID-19. For the latest report, see GAO, *COVID-19: Sustained Federal Action Is Crucial as Pandemic Enters Its Second Year,* GAO-21-387 (Washington, D.C.: Mar. 31, 2021). Our next government-wide report will be issued in July 2021 and will be available on GAO's website at https://www.gao.gov/coronavirus.

emerging infectious diseases in nursing homes, as well as CMS's response to the pandemic.

This report describes the frequency and duration of COVID-19 outbreaks in nursing homes from May 2020 through January 2021. Future GAO reports will examine more broadly infection prevention and control and emergency preparedness in nursing homes and CMS's response to the COVID-19 pandemic.

To conduct this work, we analyzed CMS and CDC data; reviewed agency guidance and documents; spoke to representatives from three national organizations that we selected because they represent nursing homes, residents, and their families; and spoke to five researchers with published research on nursing home infection control. Specifically, in our data review, we analyzed CDC data on COVID-19 reported by nursing homes from the week ending May 31, 2020, through the week ending January 31, 2021, the most recent data available at the time we conducted our review.[3] We analyzed data from 13,380 Medicare- and Medicaid-certified nursing homes that had COVID-19 data that passed CDC's and CMS's quality assurance checks in all weeks of our review period.[4] This represents approximately 88 percent of all Medicare- and Medicaid - certified nursing homes that submitted data at any point during our review period.[5]

Our analysis included multiple steps. First, we identified the nursing homes that reported at least one new COVID-19 case in a resident or staff

---

[3] The CDC data on COVID-19 in nursing homes were accessed on February 25, 2021, for the week ending January 31, 2021, from https://data.cms.gov/Covid19-nursing-home-data. Nursing homes report aggregate data to CDC on a weekly basis. According to CDC, data used in this analysis are part of a live data set, meaning that facilities can make corrections to the data at any time. The week ending May 31, 2020, is the first single week of data reported to CDC. The week ending May 24 is the only earlier week of data and could potentially include cases and deaths for multiple weeks dating back to January 1, 2020, for those homes that voluntarily reported such data. It is therefore not comparable with data for other weeks, and we excluded it.

[4] Data quality checks are performed by CDC and CMS to identify instances where facilities may have entered incorrect data, such as entering cumulative counts over time instead of new cases and other data entry errors. One thousand, eight hundred fifty-one Medicare-or Medicaid-certified nursing homes were excluded because they did not pass one or more weeks of these data quality checks during the 36 weeks of the period analyzed. These excluded homes were located in all states but one. Further, while there was variation in the percentage of homes in each state that did not pass data quality checks, no states were extreme outliers.

[5] We compared our findings to an analysis of Medicare- and Medicaid-certified nursing homes with CDC data that passed quality assurance checks in any week during our review period—rather than every week—and had similar findings.

member in any week of our review period.[6] According to CDC, a COVID-19 outbreak starts the week a nursing home reports a new COVID-19 case in a resident or staff member and ends when the nursing home has 2 consecutive weeks where they report no new staff or resident cases.[7] Using this definition of an outbreak, we determined the number and duration of outbreaks each nursing home experienced during the review period.

Next, we categorized the nursing homes with COVID-19 outbreaks into two groups based on the duration of their outbreak. So that each nursing home was represented once, we used the longest-lasting outbreak for nursing homes with more than one outbreak. We defined the groups as nursing homes with:

- Short-duration outbreaks—nursing homes with an outbreak lasting less than 5 weeks—and
- Long-duration outbreaks—that is, nursing homes with an outbreak lasting 5 or more weeks.[8]

Finally, we used CMS data to examine a selection of characteristics for nursing homes with no outbreaks, short-duration outbreaks, and long-duration outbreaks. Specifically, we examined nursing home ownership and nursing home bed size using data publicly available on CMS's website, as well as infection prevention and control deficiencies cited prior to the pandemic.[9] We used these data to describe the distribution of these characteristics and the duration of the COVID-19 outbreaks. In addition, we examined the variation among states by outbreak duration. We analyzed the CDC data as they were reported by nursing homes to CDC and publicly posted by CMS. We did not otherwise independently verify the accuracy of the information with these

---

[6] According to CDC, nursing home staff include anyone working or volunteering in the home, which includes, but is not limited to, contractors, temporary staff, or resident caregivers.

[7] See Centers for Disease Control and Prevention, *Testing Guidelines for Nursing Homes,* accessed January 13, 2021, from https://www.cdc.gov/coronavirus/2019-ncov/hcp/ nursing g-homes-testing.html#nursing-home.

[8] The cut-off point between 4 and 5 weeks for the two groups was based on the incubation period for COVID-19—which, according to CDC, is thought to extend to 2 weeks from exposure—and additional time to receive test results.

[9] Infection prevention and control deficiencies are the deficiency code used by state surveyors when a nursing home fails to meet CMS's requirements for infection prevention and control. We examined the publicly available infection prevention and control deficiencies cited in 2018 and 2019. We also analyzed data on infection prevention and control deficiencies cited from 2013 through 2017 and provided by CMS for a prior GAO report. See GAO, *Infection Control Deficiencies Were Widespread and Persistent in Nursing Homes Prior to COVID-19 Pandemic.* GAO-20-576R (Washington, D.C.: May 20, 2020).

nursing homes. We assessed the reliability of the CDC and CMS data sets used in our analyses by checking for missing values and obvious errors and reviewing relevant CDC and CMS documents. We determined the data were sufficiently reliable for the purposes of our reporting objective.

We conducted this performance audit from December 2020 to May 2021 in accordance with generally accepted government auditing standards.

Those standards require that we plan and perform the audit to obtain sufficient, appropriate evidence to provide a reasonable basis for our findings and conclusions based on our audit objectives. We believe that the evidence obtained provides a reasonable basis for our findings and conclusions based on our audit objectives.

Background

Nursing home residents are at a high risk for COVID-19 infection and death because the virus has a high mortality rate among elderly adults and those with underlying health conditions, according to CDC.[10] The congregate nature of nursing homes, with staff caring for multiple residents and residents sharing rooms and other communal spaces, as well as high incidence rates in the surrounding community, can increase the risk that COVID-19 will enter the home (for example, through staff) and easily spread.[11] Asymptomatic transmission can further complicate a nursing home's efforts to prevent and control the spread, as it allows the virus to continue to transmit in the home undetected. A growing body of evidence shows that asymptomatic transmission may be a contributing factor to nursing home COVID-19 outbreaks.[12] However, studies have shown that testing of residents and staff is

---

[10] Centers for Disease Control and Prevention, *COVID-19: People Who Live in a Nursing Home or Long-Term Care Facility,* accessed on January 5, 2021, from https://www.cdc.gov/coronavirus/2019-ncov/need-extra-precautions/people-in-nursing-homes.html.

[11] A recent study found that trends in reported COVID-19 cases among nursing home residents and staff were similar to trends in incidence of COVID-19 in surrounding communities. See S. Bagchi et al, "Rates of COVID-19 among Residents and Staff Members in Nursing Homes—United States, May 25-November 22, 2020," *Centers for Disease Control and Prevention Morbidity and Mortality Weekly Report*, January 15, 2021, vol. 70, no. 2 (2021): 52-55. From March through September 2020, CMS directed nursing homes to restrict visitors and non- essential health care personnel in nursing homes, except in certain compassionate care situations, to reduce the transmission of COVID-19.

[12] Studies have shown that approximately half of nursing home residents diagnosed with COVID-19 were asymptomatic at the time of testing. For example, see A. Kimball et al., "Asymptomatic and Presymptomatic SARS- CoV-2 Infections in Residents of a Long-

a key strategy that can allow for the timely identification and control of infections and, when paired with strict adherence to infection prevention and control practices, can be critical for containing outbreaks and protecting both residents and staff.[13]

CMS is responsible for ensuring that nursing homes meet federal quality standards to participate in the Medicare and Medicaid programs. These standards require, for example, that nursing homes establish and maintain an infection control program. To monitor compliance with these standards, CMS enters into agreements with state survey agencies in each state government to conduct inspections, including recurring comprehensive standard surveys and as-needed investigations. If a surveyor from a state survey agency determines that a nursing home violated a federal standard during a survey or investigation, the nursing home is cited for the deficiency.

We have issued several reports examining COVID-19 in nursing homes, part of our larger bodies of work on nursing home oversight and on the federal response to the COVID -19 pandemic. (See app. II for a list of related GAO products.) In May 2020, we analyzed CMS nursing home infection prevention and control deficiency data, finding that these deficiencies were widespread and persistent in nursing homes in the years prior to the COVID-19 pandemic.[14] In response to the CARES Act, we have examined the federal response to COVID-19 in nursing homes in five subsequent reports, where we reported on nursing home-related actions the Department of Health and Human Services (HHS) had taken in response to the pandemic, primarily through CMS and CDC, as well as challenges nursing homes faced responding to COVID-19. For example, in our September 2020 report we described how HHS, through CMS, implemented a COVID-19 reporting requirement for

---

Term Care Skilled Nursing Facility—King County, Washington, March 2020," *Centers for Disease Control and Prevention Morbidity and Mortality Weekly Report,* vol. 69, no. 13 (2020): 377-381; M. Arons et al., "Presymptomatic SARS-CoV-2 Infections and Transmission in a Skilled Nursing Facility," *New England Journal of Medicine*, vol. 382, no.22 (2020): 2081-2090; and S. Shi et al., "Risk Factors, Presentation, and Course of Coronavirus Disease 2019 in a Large, Academic, Long-Term Care Facility," *JAMDA*, vol. 21, no. 10 (2020): 1378-1383.

[13] See C. Telford et al., "Preventing COVID-19 Outbreaks in Long-Term Care Facilities through Preemptive Testing of Residents and Staff Members—Fulton County, Georgia, March-May 2020," *Centers for Disease Control and Prevention Morbidity and Mortality Weekly Report*, vol. 69, no. 37 (2020) 1296-1299, and J. Taylor, "Serial Testing for SARS-CoV-2 and Virus Whole Genome Sequencing Inform Infection Risk at Two Skilled Nursing Facilities with COVID-19 Outbreaks—Minnesota, April-June 2020," *Centers for Disease Control and Prevention Morbidity and Mortality Weekly Report,* vol. 69, no. 37 (2020): 1288-1295.

[14] See GAO-20-576R.

nursing homes effective May 8, 2020, and made reporting prior to May 8, 2020, optional.[15] Also in September 2020, HHS began requiring nursing homes to routinely test staff for COVID-19 based on the degree of community spread and to test staff and residents with symptoms. If a nursing home identifies a new COVID-19 case in staff or residents, all staff and residents must be tested.

Most Nursing Homes Had Multiple COVID-19 Outbreaks and 5 or More Weeks of Sustained Transmission

Our analysis of CDC data shows that, from May 2020 through January 2021, nursing homes commonly experienced multiple COVID-19 outbreaks that often lasted 5 or more weeks and were first reported in staff. This analysis highlights the challenges most nursing homes faced when responding to the COVID-19 pandemic—responding to repeated outbreaks, many with weeks of continued spread and marked by high numbers of cases and deaths. Specifically, we found that nursing homes had an average of about three outbreaks from May 2020 through January 2021, with most nursing homes (94 percent or 12,555 of the 13,380 nursing homes with CDC data that passed quality assurance checks in all weeks) experiencing more than one outbreak during our period of review.[16]

For each nursing home's longest-lasting COVID-19 outbreak, about 85 percent (11,311 nursing homes) had outbreaks lasting 5 or more weeks.[17] Conversely, for about 15 percent of nursing homes (2,005 homes), the longest outbreak was shorter in duration, lasting between 1 and 4 weeks, and 267 of

---

[15] GAO has made four recommendations to HHS related to nursing homes in our CARES Act reports, including to develop a strategy to capture more complete data on confirmed COVID-19 cases and deaths in nursing homes retroactively back to January 1, 2020. We will continue to monitor HHS's progress towards implementing these four recommendations. For the GAO CARES Act reports with nursing home-related recommendations, see GAO, COVID-19: Federal Efforts Could Be Strengthened by Timely and Concerted Actions, GAO-20-701, (Washington, D.C.: Sept. 21, 2020); COVID-19: Urgent Actions Needed to Better Ensure an Effective Federal Response, GAO-21-191, (Washington, D.C.: Nov. 30, 2020); and COVID-19: Sustained Federal Action is Crucial as Pandemic Enters its Second Year, GAO-21-387, (Washington, D.C.: March 31, 2021).

[16] Most of the remaining 6 percent of nursing homes (761 homes) had one COVID-19 outbreak while less than 1 percent (64 homes) had no outbreaks.

[17] Since many nursing homes experienced repeated COVID-19 outbreaks, we used the outbreak with the longest duration for this analysis.

those homes were able to control their outbreaks after the initial week.[18] (See Figure 1.) Further:

- Nursing homes with a long-duration outbreak also had a higher average number of resident and staff cases during the outbreak compared to nursing homes with a short-duration outbreak.
- Specifically, the average number of COVID-19 cases per outbreak for nursing homes with a long-duration outbreak was 56, while the average for nursing homes with a short-duration outbreak was 13.[19]
- For both long- and short-duration outbreaks, over half of the nursing homes (66 percent or 8,720 nursing homes) reported that these outbreaks began with a staff case the first week of the outbreak.[20]

A closer examination of the 11,311 nursing homes in the CDC data with long-duration COVID-19 outbreaks (5 or more weeks) shows the following:

- Over half of the nursing homes (61 percent or 6,858 nursing homes) had outbreaks lasting between 5 and 10 weeks. The remaining 39 percent of these homes with long-duration outbreaks (4,453 nursing homes) had outbreaks lasting more than 10 weeks. (See figure 2.)
- About one-third (36 percent or 4,045 nursing homes) had more than one long-duration outbreak during the period of our review, and 88 percent (9,921 nursing homes) also had one or more short-duration outbreaks.

---

[18] We also examined this for Medicare- and Medicaid-certified nursing homes with CDC data that passed quality assurance checks in any week during our review period—rather than every week—and found similar percentages. Specifically, for each home's longest-lasting outbreak, 12,706 of 15,231 nursing homes (83 percent) had a long-duration outbreak and 2,409 (16 percent) had a short-duration outbreak.

[19] Similarly, for the entire period of our review, total reported COVID-19 deaths for homes with long-duration outbreaks ranged from zero to 102, with an average of seven deaths per nursing home; for homes with short-duration outbreaks, deaths ranged from zero to 54, with an average of two deaths per nursing home. We analyzed deaths over the entire period of review, rather than just for the longest duration outbreak, because we cannot determine to which outbreak a death is attributed.

[20] Sixteen percent (2,095 homes) of nursing homes reported cases in residents first, and 19 percent of nursing homes (2,501 homes) reported that both residents and staff were identified with cases in the first week of the outbreak.

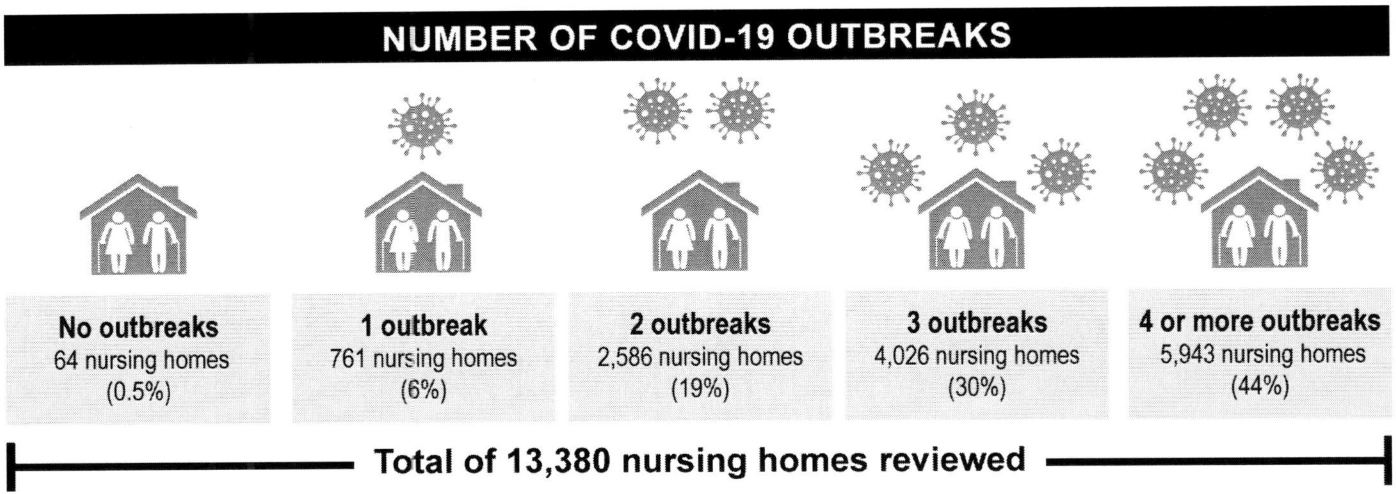

Figure 1. (Continued).

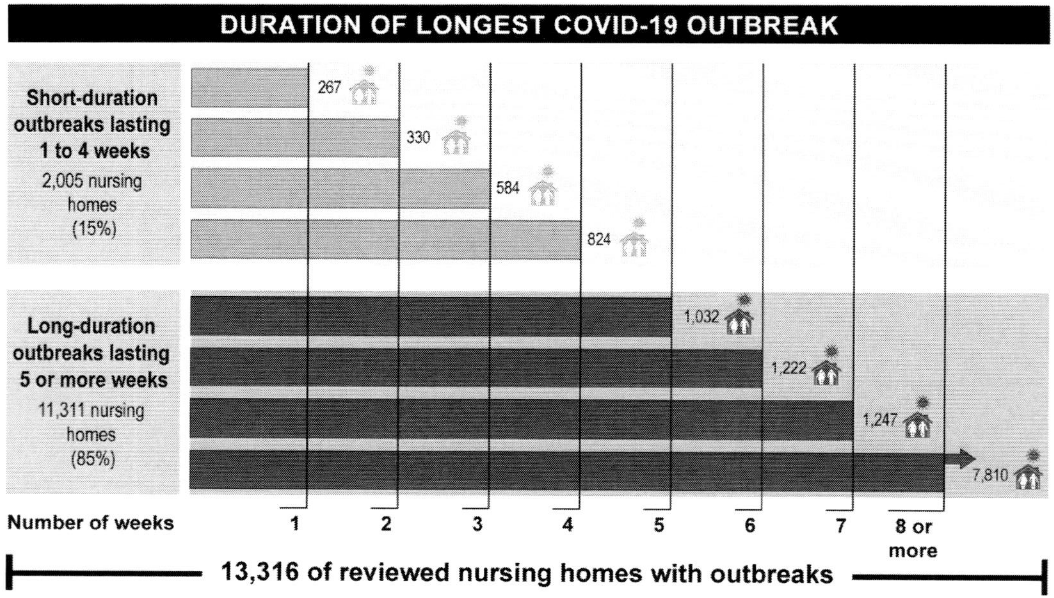

Source: GAO analysis of Centers for Disease Control and Prevention data.| GAO-21-367.

Note: The universe of 13,380 nursing homes includes Medicare- and Medicaid-certified homes with COVID-19 data that passed CDC quality assurance checks in all weeks from May 31, 2020, through January 31, 2021. An outbreak begins when a nursing home reports a new case of COVID -19 in a resident or staff member, and an outbreak ends when the nursing home has 2 consecutive weeks without a new COVID-19 case. Percentages may not add to 100 due to rounding.

Figure 1. Number and duration of COVID-19 outbreaks in nursing homes, May 31, 2020, through January 31, 2021.

- The majority of these long-duration outbreaks started between October and December 2020—generally consistent with a period of time where weekly case and death counts in nursing homes increased to their highest points since the start of the pandemic.

Further, using the CDC data and CMS nursing home data, we describe the distribution of a selection of nursing home characteristics and the duration of COVID-19 outbreaks—long-duration, short-duration, and none.

- Number of beds. We found that nursing homes with long-duration outbreaks were more likely to have a larger number of beds than homes with short-duration outbreaks. Specifically, nursing homes with less than 50 beds comprised 12 percent of all nursing homes in our review, but made up a greater share of homes with short-duration outbreaks (28 percent) and a smaller share of homes with long-duration outbreaks (9 percent). The inverse was the case for nursing homes with 100 to 199 beds, as they made up 44 percent of homes in our review overall but made up 27 percent of homes with short-duration outbreaks and 47 percent of homes with long-duration outbreaks.[21] In part, this reflects the fact that larger homes will inherently incur a higher risk of having at least one case, given that they have more residents and staff, each of whom could become that case. In addition, studies have shown that larger nursing homes with more beds and, subsequently, more residents and staff, may have a higher risk of exposure to COVID-19—particularly in areas of high community spread—and thus greater potential for more people in the facility to become infected.[22]
- Ownership. We did not see differences between the homes with long- and short-duration outbreaks and their ownership profit status (i.e., for-profit, non-profit, or government). For example, nursing homes owned by for-profit organizations, which comprised 70 percent of all nursing homes in our review, also accounted for about 70 percent of nursing homes in each of these outbreak duration groups.

---

[21] The average number of beds in the group of nursing homes with long-duration outbreaks was larger than the average number of beds in the group of nursing homes with short-duration outbreaks—an average of 110 beds compared to 77 beds. We measured number of beds using Medicare- and Medicaid-certified beds.

[22] See, for example, C. Harrington et al. "Nurse Staffing and Coronavirus Infections in California Nursing Homes," *Policy, Politics, and Nursing Practice*, vol. 21, no. 3 (2020): 174-186.

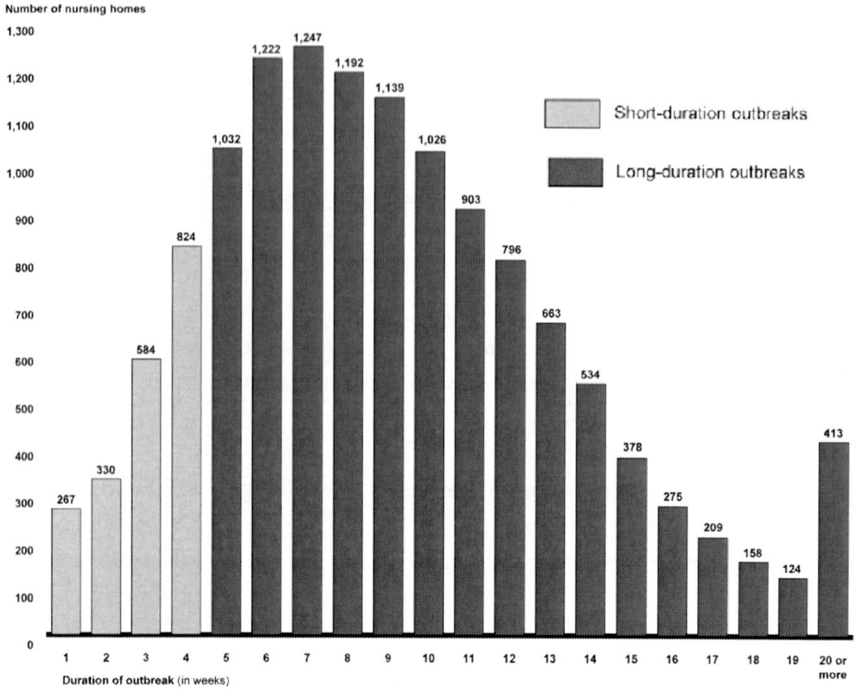

Source: GAO analysis of Centers for Disease Control and Prevention data.| GAO-21-367.

Note: The universe of 13,316 nursing homes includes Medicare- and Medicaid-certified homes with COVID-19 outbreaks and data that passed CDC quality assurance checks in all weeks from May 31, 2020, through January 31, 2021. Since many nursing homes experienced repeated COVID-19 outbreaks, we used the outbreak with the longest duration for this analysis. An outbreak begins when a nursing home reports a new case of COVID-19 in a resident or staff member, and an outbreak ends when the nursing home has 2 consecutive weeks without a new COVID-19 case.

Figure 2. Number of nursing homes by duration of longest COVID-19 outbreak, May 31, 2020, through January 31, 2021.

- History of infection prevention and control deficiencies. An examination of the distribution of nursing homes cited with infection prevention and control deficiencies prior to the pandemic (2013 through 2019) and nursing homes with long- and short-duration outbreaks did not show notable differences. This is because most nursing homes in each of these groups had infection prevention and control deficiencies cited in these years, which is consistent with our prior reporting.[23]

- Variation by state. While the precise percentage of nursing homes that had long-duration outbreaks, short-duration outbreaks, or no outbreaks varied by state, we found that in most states over three-quarters of nursing homes had long-duration outbreaks. Specifically, only eight states—Alaska, Hawaii, Maine, Massachusetts, New Hampshire, Oregon, Vermont, and Washington—had less than three-quarters of their homes with long-duration outbreaks and, therefore, had a higher combined percentage of short-duration outbreaks and homes without any outbreaks. Conversely, five states had 95 percent or more of their nursing homes that experienced long-duration outbreaks—Alabama, Arkansas, North Dakota, South Carolina, and Tennessee. (See app. I.)

Researchers and representatives of national associations and organizations we interviewed told us about several factors that can increase the risk of COVID-19 being introduced into a nursing home and spreading. These officials frequently highlighted the risks posed by a failure or inability of a nursing home to implement robust infection control practices to control the spread of the virus. For example, officials noted that once COVID-19 enters a home—which can be more likely when community transmission is high—the ability of the home to quickly test, identify, and separate infected residents and staff before they infect others is critically important to stopping the spread. In addition, officials said that a lack of personal protective equipment in the home can increase the risk of spread, because staff can become infected or infect others. Further, officials noted it can be difficult for nursing homes to adhere to infection control practices without adequate staffing. Staffing shortages can occur if staff are out due to illness, and frequent staff turnover makes it difficult for the home to ensure that new staff are trained on proper infection control practices.

John E. Dicken
Director, Health Care

---

[23] Infection prevention and control deficiencies cited by surveyors can include situations where nursing home staff did not regularly use proper hand hygiene or failed to implement preventive measures during an infectious disease outbreak, such as isolating sick residents and using masks and other personal protective equipment to control the spread of infection. See GAO-20-576R.

List of Addressees

The Honorable Patrick Leahy
Chairman

The Honorable Richard Shelby
Vice Chairman

Committee on Appropriations
United States Senate

The Honorable Ron Wyden
Chairman

The Honorable Mike Crapo
Ranking Member

Committee on Finance
United States Senate

The Honorable Patty Murray
Chairman

The Honorable Richard Burr
Ranking Member

Committee on Health, Education, Labor, and Pensions
United States Senate

The Honorable Gary C. Peters
Chairman

The Honorable Rob Portman
Ranking Member
Committee on Homeland Security and Governmental Affairs
United States Senate

The Honorable Rosa L. DeLauro
Chairwoman

The Honorable Kay Granger
Ranking Member
Committee on Appropriations
House of Representatives

The Honorable Frank Pallone, Jr.
Chairman

The Honorable Cathy McMorris Rodgers
Republican Leader

Committee on Energy and Commerce
House of Representatives

The Honorable Bennie G. Thompson
Chairman

The Honorable John Katko
Ranking Member
Committee on Homeland Security
House of Representatives

The Honorable Carolyn B. Maloney
Chairwoman

The Honorable James Comer
Ranking Member
Committee on Oversight and Reform
House of Representatives

The Honorable Richard E. Neal
Chairman

The Honorable Kevin Brady
Republican Leader
Committee on Ways and Means
House of Representatives

The Honorable Michael F. Bennet
United States Senate

Appendix I: State

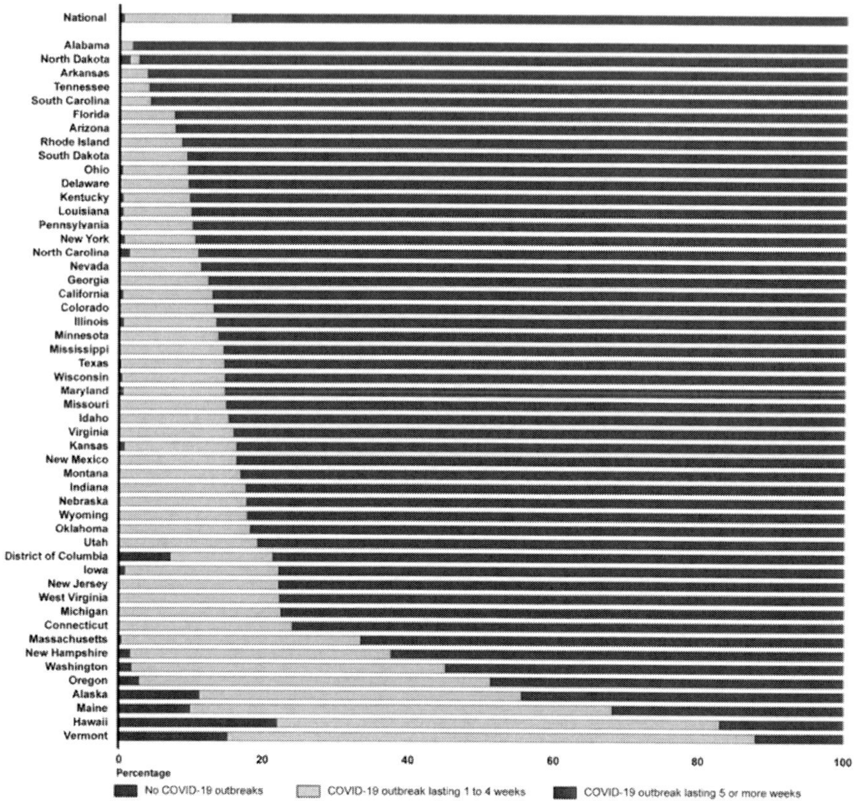

Source: GAO analysis of Centers for Disease Control and Prevention data.| GAO-21-367.

Note: The universe of 13,380 nursing homes includes Medicare- and Medicaid-certified homes with COVID-19 data that passed CDC quality assurance checks in all weeks from May 31, 2020, through January 31, 2021. Since many nursing homes experienced repeated COVID-19 outbreaks, we used the outbreak with the longest duration for this analysis. An outbreak begins when a nursing home reports a new case of COVID-19 in a resident or staff member, and an outbreak ends when the nursing home has 2 consecutive weeks without a new COVID-19 case.

Figure 3. Percentage of Nursing homes with no COVID-19 outbreaks, COVID-19 outbreaks lasting 1 through 4 weeks, and COVID-19 outbreaks lasting for 5 or more weeks, by state, May 31, 2020, through January 31, 2021.

Chapter 3

COVID-19 in Nursing Homes: Outbreak Duration Averaged 4 Weeks and Was Strongly Associated with Community Spread*

United States Government Accountability Office

Why GAO Did This Study

The COVID-19 pandemic has had a disproportionate effect on the more than 1 million residents in the nation's nursing homes. The initial unknown nature of the virus and the scope of the pandemic created unprecedented challenges. The Department of Health and Human Services, primarily through CMS and CDC, is responsible for taking steps to address COVID-19 in nursing homes, such as issuing relevant requirements and guidance.

Many studies have explored the factors associated with the presence or severity of COVID-19 in nursing homes. However, little was known about the factors associated with the duration of COVID-19 outbreaks within nursing homes.

The CARES Act directs GAO to monitor the federal pandemic response. GAO was also asked to review CMS oversight of nursing homes in light of the pandemic. This report examines how COVID-19 outbreaks affected nursing homes, and determines how nursing home factors were associated with outbreak duration.

GAO analyzed CDC and CMS nursing home data from June 2020 through December 2021, in a statistical model, and conducted a literature review.

---

* This is an edited, reformatted and augmented version of United States Government Accountability Office, Report to Congressional Addressees, Publication No. GAO-23-104291, dated December 2022.

In: COVID-19 in Nursing Homes
Editor: Fred C. Wallace
ISBN: 979-8-88697-673-1

GAO also interviewed representatives from nursing homes and state agencies from a non-generalizable sample of four states. The states were selected for variation in factors such as number of nursing home beds and COVID-19 cases.

What GAO Found

GAO analysis of data from the Centers for Disease Control and Prevention (CDC) shows that, from June 2020 through December 2021, nursing homes faced many separate COVID-19 outbreaks, with the average outbreak lasting 4 weeks. Officials GAO interviewed at six selected nursing homes in four states described a range of outbreak experiences, including critical challenges and some successes. For example, two critical challenges included:

- *Staff shortages.* Officials from five nursing homes described experiencing staffing shortages during outbreaks. For example, officials from one nursing home described a staffing crisis, noting that at one point the home was down about 25 percent of its workforce.
- *Low staff morale.* Officials from three nursing homes discussed the psychosocial effect the pandemic had on their staff and the difficulties in maintaining staff morale. For example, officials from one nursing home described how the outbreaks took away the joy of caregiving from staff, and officials believed that many staff were left traumatized.

GAO's analysis of CDC and Centers for Medicare & Medicaid Services (CMS) data found that transmission of COVID-19 in the community surrounding a nursing home, known as community spread, had the strongest association with the duration of an outbreak. Controlling for other factors, prior to the introduction of COVID-19 vaccines, nursing homes in counties experiencing low community spread had outbreaks that ended an estimated 7 days earlier than nursing homes in counties experiencing high community spread. GAO also found that most outbreaks (75 percent) began with a reported staff case during the first week. These results could indicate that, during times of higher community spread, staff have a greater likelihood of being exposed to the virus in the community and bringing it into the nursing home. Other factors GAO found that had a strong association with outbreak duration included nursing home size, reported staff shortages, and ownership type.

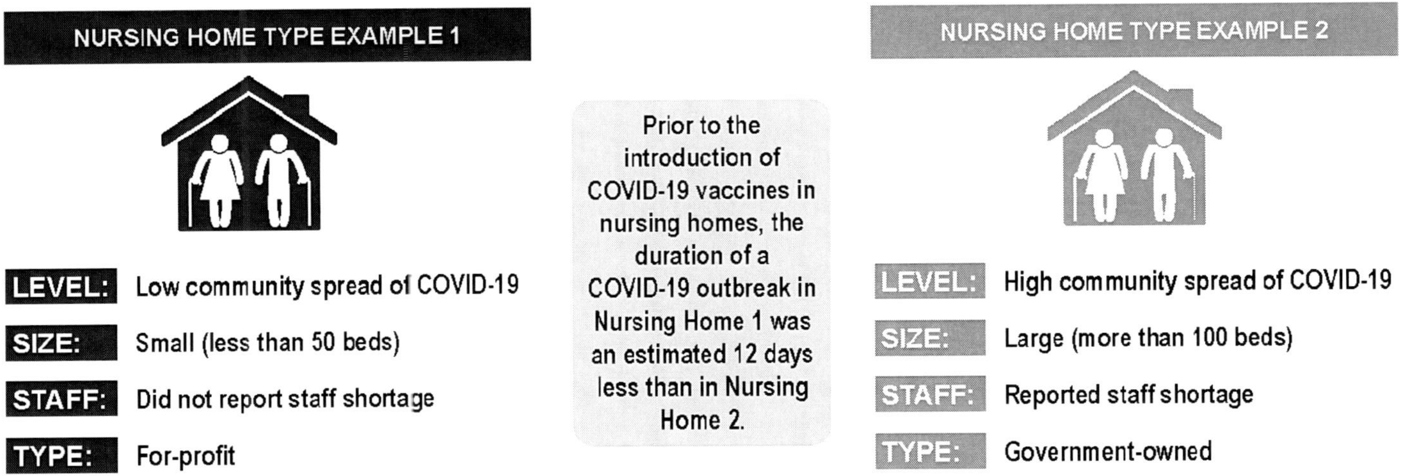

Source: GAO analysis of Centers for Disease Control and Prevention and Centers for Medicare & Medicaid Services data. | GAO-23-104291.

Note: Using multivariate statistical models, GAO estimated the association of nursing home factors, such as facility characteristics, with the likelihood that an ongoing COVID-19 outbreak would end during a given week.

GAO estimated COVID-19 outbreak duration for nursing homes with selected characteristics.

Abbreviations

CDC	Centers for Disease Control and Prevention
CMS	Centers for Medicare & Medicaid Services
HHS	Department of Health and Human Services

Letter

December 15, 2022

Congressional Addressees

COVID-19 emerged as a new and highly contagious respiratory disease that has resulted in catastrophic loss of life. These devastating consequences have been particularly pronounced for the nation's more than 1 million nursing home residents. A disproportionate share of all COVID-19 deaths reported by the Centers for Disease Control and Prevention (CDC) has been among nursing home residents.[1] The initial unknown nature of the virus that causes COVID-19, along with the scope of the pandemic, created unprecedented challenges for the state and federal agencies working to ensure the quality of care delivered in the more than 15,000 Medicare- and Medicaid-certified nursing homes.[2]

Nursing home residents are at a high risk of infection and death due to COVID-19, as older adults and those with underlying health conditions are at

---

[1] Combined nursing home resident and staff deaths from COVID-19 consistently represented about 30 percent of all COVID-19 deaths in the U.S. from May 2020 through February 2021. In May 2021, this percentage declined to about 23 percent and further decreased to about 16 percent in May 2022. See Centers for Disease Control and Prevention, *COVID Data Tracker*, accessed September 7, 2022, https://covid.cdc.gov/covid-data-tracker.

[2] Federal statutes and their implementing regulations use the terms "skilled nursing facility" (Medicare) and "nursing facility" (Medicaid). For the purposes of this report, we use the term "nursing home" to refer to both skilled nursing facilities and nursing facilities.

Medicare, the federal health insurance program for people age 65 and older, individuals under age 65 with certain disabilities, and individuals diagnosed with end-stage renal disease, covers some short-term skilled nursing and rehabilitative care for beneficiaries following an acute care hospital stay. Medicaid, a joint federal-state health program for certain low-income and medically needy individuals, is the nation's primary payer of long-term services and supports for children and adults with disabilities and aged individuals.

higher risk of severe disease.[3] In addition, the congregate nature of nursing homes, with staff caring for multiple residents and communal spaces, increases the risk that COVID-19 will easily spread. The introduction of COVID-19 vaccines in conjunction with improved infection prevention and control practices coincided with a sharp decline in nursing home cases and deaths from their initial peaks in December 2020. However, the emergence of more transmissible virus variants led to the highest resident and staff case rates in nursing homes thus far in January 2022.

While there have been several studies exploring the factors associated with the presence and severity of COVID-19 in nursing homes, little is known about the factors that are associated with the duration of outbreaks once the virus enters the home.[4]

The CARES Act includes a provision directing us to monitor the federal response to the COVID-19 pandemic.[5] Further, you asked us to examine the Centers for Medicare & Medicaid Services' (CMS) oversight of infection prevention and control protocols and the adequacy of emergency preparedness standards for emerging infectious diseases in nursing homes, as well as CMS's response to the pandemic. Since 2020, we have examined multiple aspects of the response to COVID-19 in nursing homes. Some reports are published while work on others is ongoing.[6]

This report (1) examines how COVID-19 outbreaks affected nursing homes and (2) determines how certain nursing home factors were associated with the duration of COVID-19 outbreaks.

---

[3] Centers for Disease Control and Prevention, *COVID-19: People Who Live in a Nursing Home or Long-Term Care Facility,* accessed January 5, 2021, https://www.cdc.gov/coronavirus/2019-ncov/need-extra-precautions/people-in-nursing ho mes.html.

[4] Studies have found a range of factors, such as COVID-19 transmission in the surrounding community, racial disparities, and staffing levels, that are associated with the presence or severity of COVID-19 cases and deaths in nursing homes. See appendix I for a list of such studies.

[5] Pub. L. No. 116-136, § 19010(b), 134 Stat. 281, 580 (2020). Throughout the pandemic, we regularly issued government-wide reports on the federal response to COVID-19. All government-wide reports are available on GAO's website at https://www.gao.gov/corona virus.

[6] For example, see GAO, *Infection Control Deficiencies Were Widespread and Persistent in Nursing Homes Prior to COVID-19 Pandemic*, GAO-20-576R (Washington, D.C.: May 20, 2020); *COVID-19 in Nursing Homes: Most Homes Had Multiple Outbreaks and Weeks of Sustained Transmission from May 2020 through January 2021*, GAO-21-367 (Washington, D.C.: May 19, 2021); and *COVID-19 in Nursing Homes: CMS Needs to Continue to Strengthen Oversight of Infection Prevention and Control*, GAO-22-105133 (Washington, D.C.: Sep. 14, 2022).

To understand how COVID-19 outbreaks have affected nursing homes, we analyzed CDC data on nursing home COVID-19 cases. To help inform nursing home response efforts, CDC defines the start of a COVID-19 outbreak as the week a nursing home reports a new COVID-19 case in a resident or staff member and defines the end as when the nursing home has 2 consecutive weeks where it reports no such cases.[7] Using this definition of an outbreak, we first generated descriptive statistics, including the number and duration of outbreaks each of the over 15,000 Medicare- and Medicaid-certified nursing homes experienced. We did not include the 2 consecutive weeks without a new COVID-19 case when calculating an outbreak's duration.

In addition, we interviewed state officials and nursing home officials in a non-generalizable sample of four states: California, Florida, Maryland, and Michigan. These states were selected to provide variation across: (1) geographic location; (2) number of nursing home beds; and (3) number of nursing home residents and staff with confirmed positive cases of COVID-19.[8] In each of these four states, we interviewed state survey agency and state long-term care ombudsman officials, as well as officials from at least one nursing home.[9] In total, we interviewed officials from six nursing homes that we selected to obtain variation in factors such as bed count and profit or not-for-profit status.[10] We asked nursing home officials to describe how COVID-19 outbreaks affected their nursing home, as well as to describe the challenges faced while preventing and managing COVID-19 outbreaks.

Additionally, we interviewed researchers with work related to nursing homes and COVID-19, as well as national associations with knowledge of nursing homes issues. These associations included the American Health Care Association and National Consumer Voice for Quality Long-Term Care. We

---

[7] See Centers for Disease Control and Prevention, *Interim Infection Prevention and Control Recommendations to Prevent SARS-CoV-2 Spread in Nursing Homes*, accessed April 18, 2022, https://www.cdc.gov/coronavirus/2019-ncov/hcp/long-term-care.html.

[8] Nursing home characteristics data were as of June 2020, and COVID-19 case rates were as of November 1, 2020.

[9] CMS enters into agreements with survey agencies in each state (known as state survey agencies) to monitor compliance with federal quality of care standards by conducting both recurring comprehensive standard surveys (inspections) and as-needed investigations.
Under the federal Older Americans Act, every state is required to have an Ombudsman Program that addresses complaints and advocates for improvements in the long-term care system, including nursing homes, as a condition of receiving funds under the act.

[10] We conducted the original interviews from December 2020 through August 2021 and followed up with officials at each state survey agency, state long-term care ombudsman, and nursing home from November 2021 through March 2022.

discussed with researchers and association representatives the challenges faced by nursing homes during the pandemic.

To determine how certain nursing home factors were associated with the duration of COVID-19 outbreaks, we analyzed CMS data on nursing home staffing levels, resident demographics, and facility characteristics; CDC data on county-level COVID-19 community transmission levels and nursing home COVID-19 cases; and Health Resources and Services Administration data on county-level metropolitan, micropolitan, and rural designations. We developed multivariate statistical models to determine the significance of each selected factor in estimating the probability of an outbreak ending at any given week from June 14, 2020, through January 2, 2022 (the last full week of the 2021 calendar year).

Specifically, our statistical models controlled for the transmission levels of COVID-19 in the surrounding community, several nursing home characteristics, several measures of nursing home staffing levels, and several other factors, including prior infection prevention and control deficiencies. We could not control for all factors that may affect outbreak duration, such as state and local COVID-19 policies, local compliance with those policies, or nursing home adherence to infection prevention and control practices. Therefore, our model provides information on possible associations in the data and does not establish a causal relationship between the factors and outbreak duration.

To provide context to these findings, we conducted a literature review to determine what is known about the factors associated with COVID-19 outbreaks in nursing homes and identified 40 pertinent studies, which we reviewed. For a description of our literature review methodology and its findings, see appendix I.

We assessed the reliability of the various data sets we used by reviewing relevant CDC, CMS, and Health Resources and Services Administration data documentation, interviewing knowledgeable agency officials, and performing tests of the data to identify any outliers or anomalies. We determined that these datasets were sufficiently reliable for the purposes of our reporting objectives. For additional information about our descriptive and statistical analyses and model, see appendix II.

We conducted this performance audit from April 2020 to December 2022 in accordance with generally accepted government auditing standards. Those standards require that we plan and perform the audit to obtain sufficient, appropriate evidence to provide a reasonable basis for our findings and conclusions based on our audit objectives. We believe that the evidence obtained provides a reasonable basis for our findings and conclusions based on our audit objectives.

Background

The Department of Health and Human Services (HHS), primarily through CMS and CDC, has led the response to the COVID-19 pandemic in nursing homes. CMS is the federal oversight agency responsible for ensuring that nursing homes meet federal quality standards to be eligible to participate in the Medicare and Medicaid programs.[11] CDC issues guidance with recommendations for preventing and managing infectious diseases and operates infectious disease surveillance systems. CDC also provides technical assistance through programs aimed at supporting and assessing infection prevention and control in nursing homes, and tracking infection prevention and control data.[12]

The COVID-19 pandemic has had a disproportionate effect on nursing home residents thus far. Nursing home residents are at a high risk of infection and death due to COVID-19, as older adults and those with underlying health conditions are at a higher risk of severe disease. In addition, the congregate nature of nursing homes increases the risk of transmission.[13] We have previously reported on a number of COVID-19 issues in nursing homes, including challenges nursing homes have faced and the number and duration of outbreaks early in the pandemic. For example, our past work found that

---

[11] To monitor compliance with these standards, CMS enters into agreements with survey agencies in each state to conduct recurring comprehensive standard surveys and as- needed investigations. Beginning in March 2020, CMS required state survey agencies to conduct focused infection control surveys, a new type of survey in response to the pandemic with a narrower scope than a standard survey, for 20 percent of nursing homes in their state annually, prioritizing those facilities that report new COVID-19 cases and low vaccination rates. If a state survey agency determines that a nursing home violated a federal standard, the nursing home is cited for the deficiency.

[12] According to CDC officials, this includes developing resources to support implementation of prevention and surveillance activities, conducting and supporting onsite and remote infection prevention and control assessments, and supporting outbreak field investigations.

[13] According to CDC, COVID-19 is spread in three main ways: (1) breathing in small droplets or particles exhaled by an infected person; (2) having these small droplets and particles land on the eyes, nose, or mouth, especially through a cough or a sneeze; and (3) touching eyes, nose, or mouth with hands that have the virus on them. See Centers for Disease Control and Prevention, *How COVID-19 Spreads*, accessed April 16, 2022, https://www.cdc.gov/coronavirus/2019-ncov/prevent-getting-sick/how-covid-spreads.html.

most nursing homes had multiple outbreaks and weeks of sustained COVID-19 transmission from May 2020 through January 2021.[14]

Many studies have explored the factors associated with the presence or severity of COVID-19 in nursing homes, finding a range of associated factors, such as COVID-19 in the surrounding community, nursing home size, and racial disparities. For example, several studies all found that nursing homes with fewer beds were associated with less severe outbreaks.[15]

The duration of an outbreak within a nursing home is also important as it may indicate how well a nursing home can control the spread of the virus, as well as having implications related to staffing needs, space constraints, and resident well-being. For example, CDC guidance recommends a nursing home maintain dedicated space for residents with confirmed infections during a COVID-19 outbreak, if possible.[16] This can require additional nursing staff and strain a home's available space and resources. In addition, in March 2020, CMS released guidance restricting visitation and suspending group dining and activities to prevent the spread of the virus. Initially these restrictions were at all times; starting in September 2020, visitation was restricted only during active COVID-19 outbreaks.[17] These restrictions had unintended

---

[14] For challenges, see, for example, GAO, *COVID-19: Urgent Actions Needed to Better Ensure an Effective Federal Response*, GAO-21-191 (Washington, D.C.: Nov. 30, 2020). For number and duration of outbreaks, see GAO, *COVID-19 in Nursing Homes: Most Homes Had Multiple Outbreaks and Weeks of Sustained Transmission from May 2020 through January 2021*, GAO-21-367 (Washington, D.C.: May 19, 2021).

[15] See appendix I. For example, Elizabeth M. White et al., "Variation in SARS-CoV-2 Prevalence in U.S. Skilled Nursing Facilities," *Journal of the American Geriatrics Society*, vol. 68, no. 10 (2020): 2167-2173, and Sheryl Zimmerman, et al., "Nontraditional Small House Nursing Homes Have Fewer COVID-19 Cases and Deaths," *JAMDA*, vol. 22, no. 3 (2021): 489-493.

[16] CDC guidance specifies that staff assigned to the COVID-19 unit only work in this unit when it is in use and that, at a minimum, such staff include the primary nursing assistants and nurses assigned to care for these residents. See Centers for Disease Control and Prevention, *Interim Infection Prevention and Control Recommendations to Prevent SARS- CoV-2 Spread in Nursing Homes*, accessed July 24, 2022, https://www.cdc.gov/coronavirus/2019-ncov/hcp/long-term-care.html.

[17] CMS initially restricted visitation and suspended group dining and activities in March 2020. After the initial restrictions, CMS changed its guidance multiple times—in September 2020, March 2021, and April 2021—to allow for more visitation and group activities, while identifying some situations where limitations would be appropriate. In November 2021, all visitation limitations were fully lifted. See Centers for Medicare & Medicaid Services, *Guidance for Infection Control and Prevention of COVID-19 in Nursing Homes*, QSO-20-14-NH, (Baltimore, Md.: March 13, 2020) and Centers for Medicare & Medicaid Services, *Nursing Home Visitation – COVID-19*, QSO-20-39-NH, (Baltimore, Md.: Sept. 17, 2020), revised March 10, 2021, April 27, 2021, and November 12, 2021.

consequences on residents, such as isolation and declining health.[18] The longer a nursing home is responding to a COVID-19 outbreak, the longer staff and residents face these issues. However, we found that little was known about the factors that contribute to the length of outbreaks once the virus enters the home.[19]

CMS has required that nursing homes report COVID-19 information weekly to CDC, including resident and staff case and death counts, since May 2020.[20] CDC data show that, for the week ending May 31, 2020, through the end of 2020, there were fluctuations in new weekly confirmed cases among residents and staff. The introduction of vaccines in nursing homes at the end of December 2020, in conjunction with improved infection prevention and control practices, was a key turning point when cases and deaths began to decline. COVID-19 nursing home cases and deaths remained low through the first part of 2021, but, from the summer of 2021 through the end of that calendar year (coinciding with the emergence of the COVID-19 Delta variant), nursing home cases began to rise. Then, in January 2022 (coinciding with the emergence of the COVID-19 Omicron variant), cases in residents and staff quickly jumped to levels far exceeding the peak seen prior to the introduction of COVID-19 vaccines.[21]

---

[18] We have reported on the worsening of several key indicators of nursing home resident mental and physical health during 2020 and 2021. Nursing home officials and national organizations attributed this worsening in part to the isolation residents experienced. See GAO, *COVID-19 in Nursing Homes: CMS Needs to Continue to Strengthen Oversight of Infection Prevention and Control*, GAO-22-105133 (Washington, D.C: Sept. 14, 2022).

[19] One study in our literature review examined the number of weeks a nursing home was in the top decile of the national distribution of weekly confirmed resident COVID-19 cases, which is described as the persistence of the outbreak. The study found that nursing home quality ratings were associated with COVID-19 persistence. See Christianna S. Williams, et al., "The association of nursing home quality ratings and spread of COVID-19," *Journal of the American Geriatrics Society*, vol. 69, no. 8 (2021): 2070-2078.

[20] 42 C.F.R. § 483.80(g) (2021).

[21] According to CDC, viruses, such as the virus that causes COVID-19, constantly change through mutation, and new variants are expected to occur. The Delta variant became the dominant COVID-19 strain circulating in the U.S. during the week ending July 3, 2021. The Omicron variant superseded the Delta variant to become the dominant COVID-19 strain circulating in the U.S. during the week ending December 25, 2021. As of April 5, 2022, CDC has reported the presence of multiple sublineages of the Omicron variant in the U.S., including BA.2; BA.2 became the dominant strain circulating in the U.S. during the week ending March 26, 2022.

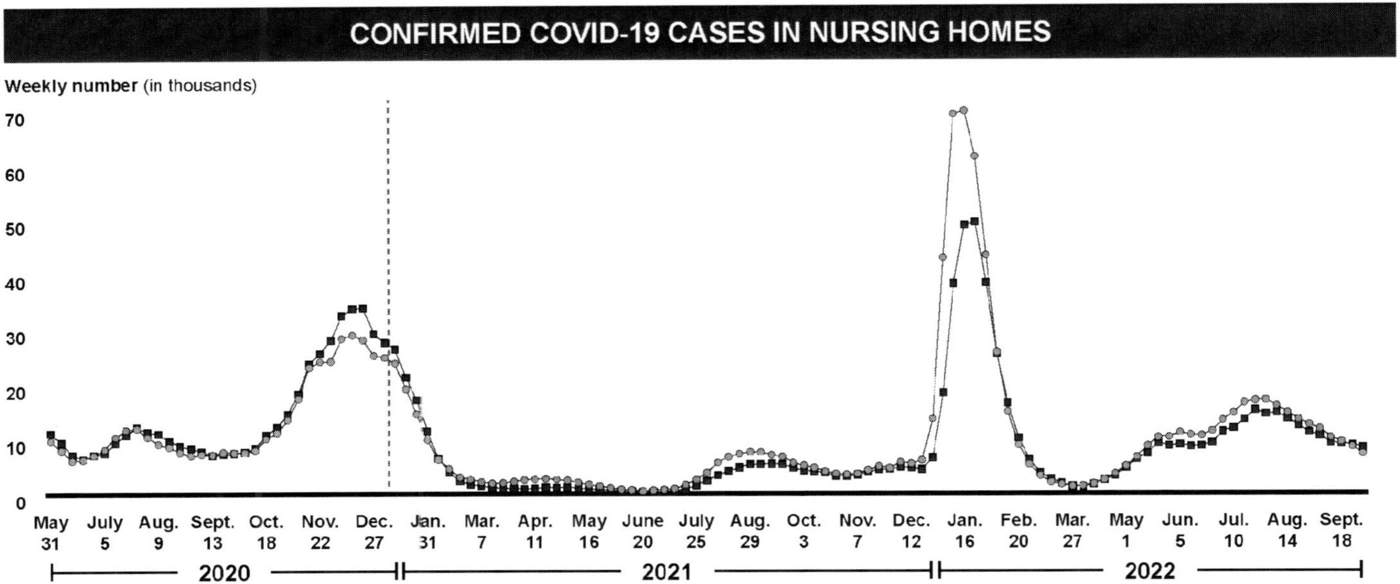

Figure 1. (Continued).

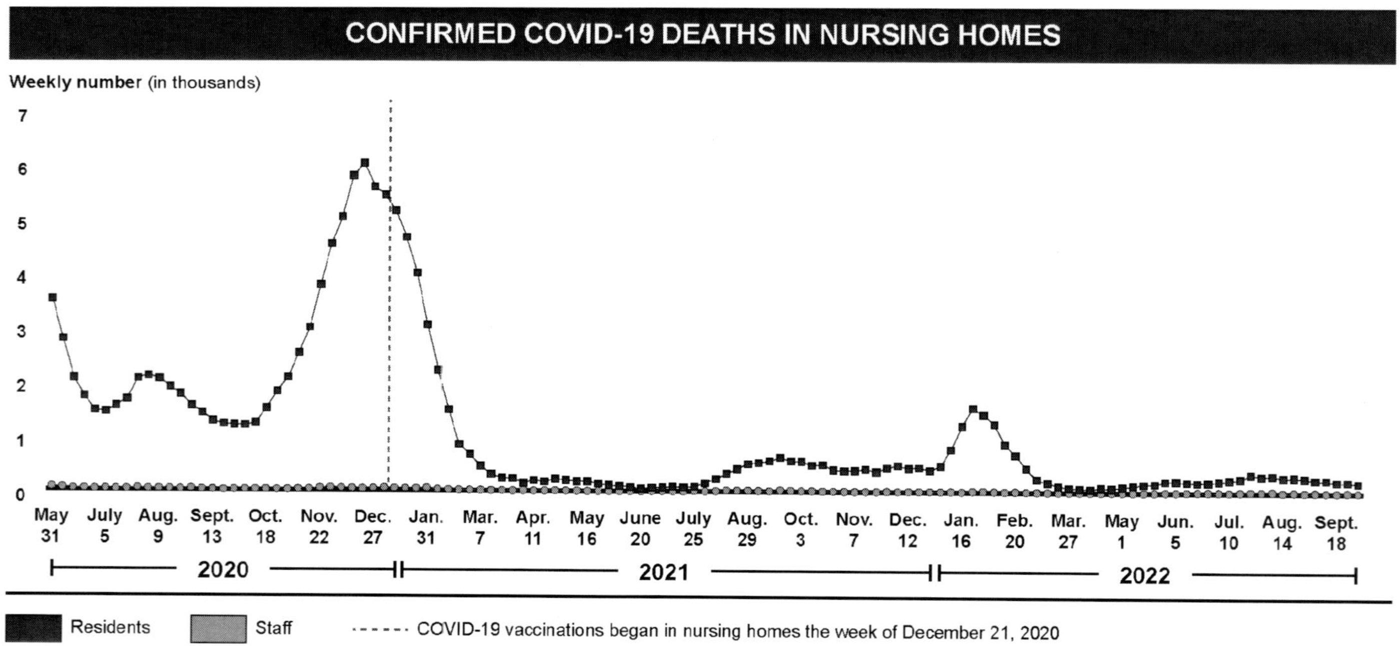

Source: GAO analysis of Centers for Disease Control and Prevention (CDC) data. | GAO-23-104291.

Figure 1. New weekly confirmed COVID-19 cases and deaths among U.S. nursing home residents and staff, weeks ending May 31, 2020, through October 2, 2022.

However, COVID-19 deaths have not risen at the same rate during these more recent peaks in cases, likely due to protection from severe illness and death provided by vaccines.[22] See Figure 1.[23]

Nursing Home COVID-19 Outbreaks Lasted 4 Weeks on Average and Selected Nursing Homes Described a Range of Outbreak Experiences

From June 14, 2020, through January 2, 2022, nursing home COVID-19 outbreaks lasted an average of 4 weeks.[24] Officials we interviewed at six selected nursing homes described a range of experiences during such outbreaks, including many challenges and some areas of success.

Nursing Homes Experienced Many COVID-19 Outbreaks from June 2020 through December 2021 with the Average Outbreak Lasting 4 Weeks

Nursing homes experienced many COVID-19 outbreaks from June 14, 2020, through January 2, 2022, with the average outbreak lasting 4 weeks. Specifically, the 15,281 nursing homes in our analysis experienced from one

[22] As of May 1, 2022, according to CDC data, nursing homes reported that 88.2 percent of residents and 89.7 percent of staff had a complete vaccination—meaning the resident had received all doses required to be fully vaccinated (two doses of a two-dose mRNA series or one dose of a single-dose vaccine). Additionally, nursing homes reported that 80.6 percent of residents and 53.2 percent of staff had received an additional primary or booster dose of the vaccine.

[23] Dates refer to the end of a week (e.g., May 31, 2020, refers to the entire week from May 25, 2020, through May 31, 2020).

According to CDC, data used in this figure are part of a live data set, meaning that facilities can correct the data at any time. This figure reflects data downloaded as of October 24, 2022, and includes data through the week ending October 2, 2022. We excluded data for the week ending May 24, 2020, because it is the first week for which data are available and includes cases and deaths from multiple weeks dating back to January 1, 2020.

Weekly case and death counts are likely underreported because they do not include data for the nursing homes that did not report COVID-19 data to CDC for that week or from nursing homes that submitted data that failed data quality assurance checks. Additionally, CMS does not require nursing homes to report data prior to May 2020, although nursing homes may do so voluntarily.

[24] An outbreak begins when a nursing home reports a new case of COVID-19 in a resident or staff member, and an outbreak ends when the nursing home has 2 consecutive weeks without a new COVID-19 case. The outbreak duration does not include the 2 consecutive weeks without a new COVID-19 case.

to 16 outbreaks, with an average of 7.6 outbreaks and a total of 102,992 outbreaks across all homes during our period of review.[25] The average outbreak duration was 4 weeks, ranging from 1 week (42 percent of total outbreaks) to 53 weeks (less than 1 percent of total outbreaks). While shorter outbreaks were more common, nearly all nursing homes (13,898 of 15,281 nursing homes, or 91 percent) experienced at least one longer-lasting outbreak of 5 or more weeks.[26] (See Figure 2). This illustrates how nursing homes were heavily affected by the COVID-19 pandemic—requiring nursing home staff to respond to, and residents to experience, repeated outbreaks and weeks of continued spread of the virus.

We found that the average duration of COVID-19 outbreaks beginning near the end of both 2020 and 2021 were longer than outbreaks beginning at other points in either year. Specifically, the longest average outbreaks began in November 2020 and December 2021, lasting an average of 7 weeks and ranging from 1 to 32 weeks and from 1 to 17 weeks, respectively. (See Figure 3). These trends follow a similar pattern to the trends seen in the number of COVID-19 cases reported in nursing homes over the same periods. There were spikes in cases in late 2020, prior to the availability of vaccines in nursing homes, and at the beginning of 2022, corresponding with the emergence of the initial COVID-19 Omicron variant. However, the increases in average outbreak duration appear to precede the spikes in case numbers reported in nursing homes by approximately 1 month. This may be because any outbreaks beginning before the spike in cases continued to spread due to the growing caseloads.

High rates of COVID-19 in the community surrounding a nursing home can increase the risk that the virus will enter the home (for example, through staff or visitors) and could spread. We found that nursing homes reported that most outbreaks began with a staff case.[27]

---

[25] During our period of review, 25 nursing homes reported zero COVID-19 outbreaks.

[26] We previously reported that, from May 2020 through January 2021—a shorter period of review than this analysis—most nursing homes had multiple COVID-19 outbreaks (with an average of about three outbreaks), and 85 percent of homes had outbreaks lasting 5 or more weeks. See GAO-21-367.

[27] Our calculation is based on data reported by nursing homes to CDC on a weekly basis. We do not take into account how many staff or residents were infected during the week, but just identify which category was reported first. Multiple contagion lines are possible for any outbreak, including contagion lines that were not detected by the testing regiment in place at the time.

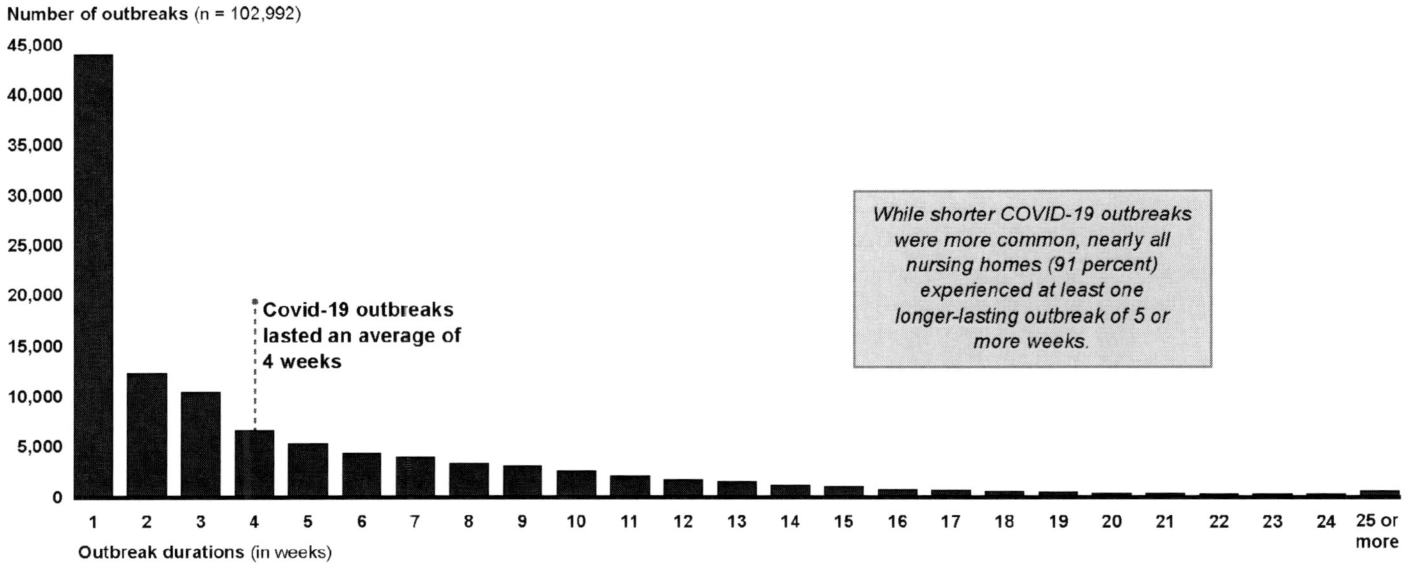

Source: GAO analysis of Centers for Disease Control and Prevention data. | GAO-23-104291.

Note: An outbreak begins when a nursing home reports a new case of COVID-19 in a resident or staff member, and an outbreak ends when the nursing home has 2 consecutive weeks without a new COVID-19 case. The outbreak duration does not include the 2 consecutive weeks without a new COVID-19 case.

Figure 2. Duration of COVID-19 outbreaks in nursing homes, June 14, 2020, through January 2, 2022.

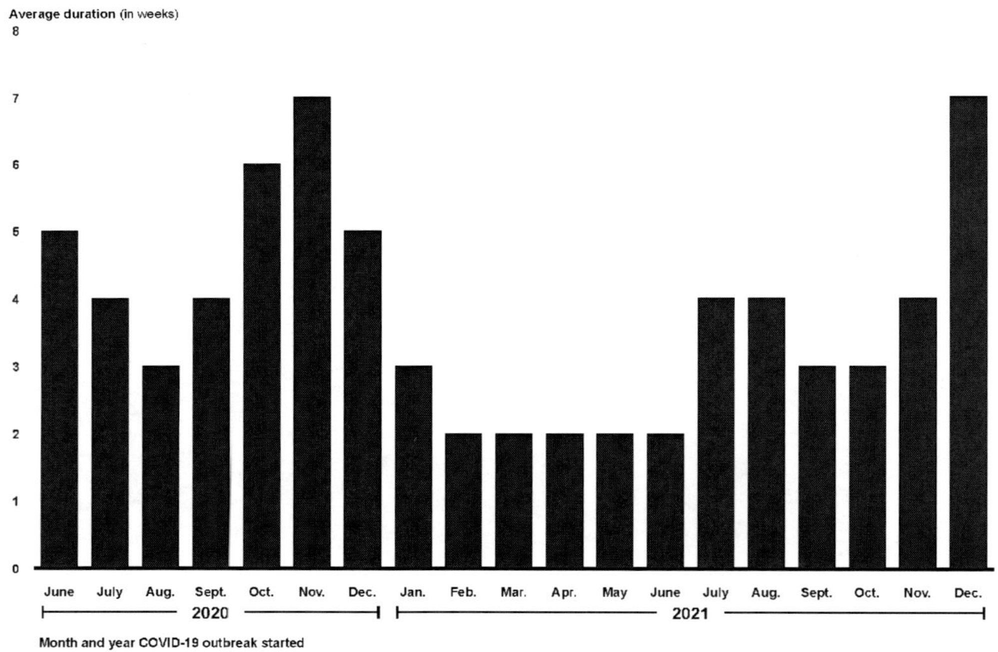

Source: GAO analysis of Centers for Disease Control and Prevention data. | GAO-23-104291.

Note: An outbreak begins when a nursing home reports a new case of COVID-19 in a resident or staff member, and an outbreak ends when the nursing home has 2 consecutive weeks without a new COVID-19 case. The outbreak duration does not include the 2 consecutive weeks without a new COVID-19 case.

Figure 3. Average duration of COVID-19 outbreaks in nursing homes by month the outbreak began, June 14, 2020 through January 2, 2022.

Specifically, 74.9 percent of all outbreaks began with a reported staff case the first week of the outbreak, 12.0 percent began with a reported resident case, and 13.1 percent began with both a reported staff and resident case.[28]

Nursing Homes Described a Range of Outbreak Experiences, Noting Challenges and Successes

Officials at the six nursing homes we interviewed described a range of experiences during their COVID-19 outbreaks. In describing their experiences, the nursing home officials highlighted a number of challenges as well as successes when discussing how they prevented and managed outbreaks. See Table 1 for a summary of each nursing home's experience with COVID-19 outbreaks. For more information on these nursing homes' experiences during outbreaks, see Appendix III.

Table 1. Nursing home officials' descriptions of COVID-19 outbreaks

Nursing home	Nursing home officials' descriptions of COVID-19 outbreaks
Nursing home A	This nursing home's first case was a staff member in July 2020, and it was caught early. The required biweekly COVID-19 testing caught additional staff cases throughout the pandemic. The nursing home's first resident outbreak was in October 2020 and started with five residents and then spread to an additional 16 residents. The nursing home officials believed that COVID-19 entered the home from a resident who left the home regularly for dialysis. A year later, in October 2021, the home had a second major resident outbreak.
Nursing home B	This nursing home experienced its largest outbreak in December 2021 with the Omicron surge. During this time, 20 percent of its residents and staff tested positive. Officials attributed this outbreak in part to the re-opening of visitation that occurred in November 2021. Prior to the outbreak, the home had only seen a few cases at a time, and its COVID-19-positive residents had avoided severe illness.
Nursing home C	Officials from this nursing home said that it kept COVID-19 out of the facility until May 2020. The first of two resident outbreaks started with a few staff contracting COVID-19 from the community. Soon after, two residents tested positive, then two more, and so on. During the first outbreak, the virus spread slowly, but the second outbreak in late 2020 spread more rapidly—from two residents to 10 or 12 residents almost immediately.

[28] This is consistent with our prior reporting where we found that 66 percent of all nursing homes from May 2020 through January 2021 reported that their longest-lasting COVID-19 outbreak started with a reported staff case the first week of the outbreak. See GAO-21-367.

Table 1. (Continued)

Nursing home D	Early in 2020, a COVID-19 outbreak affected about a dozen residents. The nursing home's second outbreak in the fall of 2020 was very hard on residents and staff, with 40 residents dying. Officials believed the virus entered the facility through staff as, at the time, the home's staff and the surrounding community had low vaccination rates. In addition to the emotional toll on residents and staff, the number of resident deaths plus staff attrition resulted in the nursing home losing about 50 percent of its capacity and closing a sister nursing home.
Nursing home E	Officials from this nursing home said that it kept COVID-19 out of the facility until July 2020. The outbreak lasted about 5 weeks and culminated with 32 of about 70 residents and 12 staff infected. Eight of those residents died. After that outbreak, the nursing home did not experience any additional large outbreaks, only a few isolated cases. Officials could not trace the origin of the outbreak, but believed that COVID-19 was brought into the facility by a staff member.
Nursing home F	Early in the pandemic, this nursing home had some staff members test positive, but COVID-19 was not transferred to the residents. The first resident did not test positive until November 2020. Officials believed that it was brought into the facility by staff. The home had another outbreak in January 2021 and was able to contain COVID-19 to just one floor of their three-floor facility for a time, but eventually the virus spread.

Source: GAO interviews with officials from selected nursing homes in four states. | GAO-23-104291.

While describing their experiences with COVID-19 outbreaks, officials from all six selected nursing homes highlighted a number of critical challenges their homes faced. Specifically, the challenges they described included staffing issues, physical and psychosocial effects on residents, physical space constraints, and supply issues.

- *Staffing issues.* Officials from five of the six nursing homes described challenges related to staffing, including staffing shortages and issues with maintaining staff morale. In addition, the long-term care ombudsman and state survey agency officials in all four selected states also highlighted issues around insufficient staffing, particularly how it can negatively affect resident care.[29]
    - *Staff shortages.* Officials from five of the six nursing homes described experiencing staff shortages during COVID-19

[29] For example, one long-term care state ombudsman described that, because of staffing shortages, staff were only able to address the basic needs of residents, which has resulted in reports of an increase in pressure sores and other issues of resident neglect. Another state long-term care ombudsman described resident concerns of having insufficient staff to meet their needs, where residents of one nursing home described being left on the toilet or bedpan for an hour waiting for staff assistance.

outbreaks.[30] For example, Nursing Home A officials described a staffing "crisis," noting that at one point the home lost about 25 full-time employees, an approximately 25 percent reduction in workforce. Nursing Home E officials described losing about half of its staff, which resulted in the closing of a section of the home and a reliance on traveling nurses and certified nurse assistants to replenish its workforce. Nursing Home F officials noted that, with such limited staff, they had to make difficult choices, including moving the remaining staff between COVID-19 and non-COVID- 19 units, which increased the risk of spreading the virus to uninfected residents. Further, Nursing Home D officials explained that being located in a rural area meant that they had fewer available staff, which sometimes resulted in "scary" staffing shortages.

- *Staff morale.* Officials from three of the six nursing homes discussed the psychosocial effect the pandemic had on their staff and the difficulties in maintaining staff morale. For example, Nursing Home D officials described how the outbreaks took away from staff the joy of caregiving and felt that many staff were left traumatized. In addition, Nursing Home B officials found it difficult to find staff willing to work in the COVID-19 units due to the risk of exposure to the virus.

- *Physical and psychosocial effects on residents.* Officials from five of the six nursing homes described challenges with balancing the costs and benefits of nursing home visitation restrictions and other changes to resident rights.[31] While visitation restrictions may have helped prevent or mitigate the spread of COVID-19 in nursing homes,

[30] In September 2020 we reported that, as of July 26, 2020, CDC data showed that 18 percent of nursing homes were reporting a shortage of aides, about 16 percent were reporting a shortage of nursing staff, about 9 percent were reporting a shortage of other staff, and 2 percent were reporting a shortage of clinical staff. These shortages persisted over time. See GAO, *COVID-19: Federal Efforts Could Be Strengthened by Timely and Concerted Actions*, GAO-20-701 (Washington, D.C.: Sept. 21, 2020), 131; *COVID-19: Urgent Actions Needed to Better Ensure an Effective Federal Response*, GAO-21-191 (Washington, D.C.: Nov. 30, 2020), 68; *COVID-19: Critical Vaccine Distribution, Supply Chain, Program Integrity, and Other Challenges Require Focused Federal Attention*, GAO-21-265 (Washington, D.C.: Jan. 28, 2021), 64; and *COVID-19: Sustained Federal Action Is Crucial as Pandemic Enters Its Second Year*, GAO-21-387 (Washington, D.C.: Mar. 31, 2021), 77.

[31] These challenges are consistent with our prior reporting, which found worsening mental and physical health indicators among nursing home residents during the first year of the pandemic. See GAO-22-105133.

interviewees highlighted the physical and psychosocial harm that these restrictions caused for residents and families. For example, Nursing Home C officials noted that the home relies heavily on social interaction, so, even more than visitation, the suspension of dining facility activities resulted in declines in resident physical and mental health. Specifically, the staff began to see unplanned resident weight loss and an increased need for anti-depressant drugs. Officials told us many of the residents just "gave up." All four selected states' long-term care ombudsmen and two of the four states' survey agencies also highlighted this challenge.[32]

- *Physical space constraints.* Officials from five of the six nursing homes described how the nursing homes' physical space limited their ability to comply with COVID-19 infection control guidelines. For example, Nursing Home E officials explained that, in order to isolate COVID-19-positive residents, the home had to shuffle healthy residents from one room to another, which may have unintentionally spread the virus. In addition, Nursing Home C officials described how they had to keep expanding the boundaries of the COVID-19 unit as more and more residents were diagnosed with the virus. Among the four selected states, one long-term care ombudsmen and officials from two state survey agencies also noted this challenge.[33]
- *Supply issues.* Officials from five of the six nursing homes discussed difficulty acquiring sufficient personal protective equipment early in the pandemic.[34] Officials at Nursing Home E explained that the limited supply of N95 respirators exacerbated an outbreak in July 2020, as many residents and some staff had to use regular procedure masks instead, which are not as protective against the virus. Three

---

[32] One state long-term care ombudsman said that her staff had witnessed loneliness, weight loss, and significant cognitive declines among residents they had known prior to the pandemic; the official said that residents who had previously recognized ombudsmen staff now looked at them "shell-shocked and blank." Another state's long-term care ombudsman said that some residents appeared to have aged 10 years over a 2- or 3- month time period.

[33] Officials at the two state survey agencies said that the physical layout and aging infrastructure of nursing homes made it difficult to establish separate COVID-19 zones and isolation rooms.

[34] This is consistent with our prior reporting on nursing home supply shortages during the COVID-19 pandemic. For example, in September 2020 we reported that, as of July 26, 2020, CDC data showed that 22 percent of nursing homes were reporting that they did not have a 1-week supply of one or more types of personal protective equipment (N95 respirators, surgical masks, gloves, eye protection, or gowns). However, as we reported in January 2021, by December 6, 2020, this number had decreased to 10 percent of nursing homes. See GAO-20-701, 129; GAO-21-191, 67; and GAO-21-265, 63.

selected states' long-term care ombudsmen and officials at all four states' survey agencies also described this as a challenge early in the pandemic.[35]

While describing their experiences with COVID-19 outbreaks, officials from five of the six nursing homes we interviewed also noted some areas of success. For example, officials from three nursing homes described having success early in the pandemic preventing COVID-19 from entering the home. Nursing Home B officials attributed their early success to county actions that resulted in low levels of COVID-19 in the community surrounding the nursing home. Specifically, Nursing Home B is located in an isolated area and the county decided to close roads into the area to keep travelers out. Nursing Homes A and C officials discussed proactive measures that they took to prevent COVID-19, such as suspending new admissions, restricting residents to their rooms, and adopting face mask requirements. However, ultimately, all six selected nursing homes had COVID-19 outbreaks.

Transmission of COVID-19 in the Surrounding Community Had the Strongest Association with Outbreak Duration in Nursing Homes

Based on our analyses, we determined that transmission of COVID-19 in the community surrounding a nursing home—known as community spread—had the strongest association with the duration of an outbreak in the home, followed by the size of the nursing home, whether the nursing home reported staff shortages, and the type of nursing home ownership.[36] Specifically, prior

---

[35] One state long-term care ombudsman described how residents could not get the therapy they needed as providers would not come in to a home that lacked adequate personal protective equipment.

[36] These factors were statistically significant at a p-value less than 0.05 and had a significant effect on the probability of an outbreak ending in a given week, which we defined as at least plus or minus 1 day (parameter estimate of at least plus or minus 0.14) in either one of the two models. We created two models—one for prior to the introduction of COVID-19 vaccines in nursing homes and one for after the introduction of vaccines in nursing homes. Additional factors were also statistically significant at a p-value less than 0.05, but their impact on outbreak duration was smaller. See Table 9 in appendix II for a list of all factors analyzed.
CDC COVID-19 community transmission levels—high, substantial, moderate, or low—describe the amount of COVID-19 spread within each county based on the total new cases per 100,000 persons within the last 7 days and the percentage of positive diagnostic and screening nucleic acid amplification tests during the last 7 days. Health care facilities use these

to the introduction of COVID-19 vaccines, being a small, for-profit nursing home that did not report staffing shortages and was located in a county experiencing low community spread was associated with a higher probability of a COVID-19 outbreak ending roughly 12 days earlier when compared to a large, government-owned nursing home that reported staff shortages and was located in a county experiencing high community spread.

Using multivariate statistical models, we estimated the association of nursing home factors with the likelihood that an ongoing COVID-19 outbreak would end during a given week over two different time periods— prior to the introduction of COVID-19 vaccines in nursing homes and after the introduction of vaccines in nursing homes.[37] Generally, the magnitude of the association of a given factor on outbreak duration was lower in the period after the introduction of vaccines compared to the period prior to the introduction of vaccines.[38] This was the case for community spread, nursing home size, and nursing home-reported staff shortages, but to varying degrees.

Community Spread

Community spread of COVID-19 had the strongest association with the duration of an outbreak in a nursing home throughout our period of review. Specifically, we found that nursing homes located in counties experiencing low, moderate, or substantial levels of community spread had a higher probability of their outbreaks ending during a given week— meaning their

---

transmission levels to determine infection control interventions. This is unique from CDC COVID-19 community levels, which the agency recommends that individuals and communities use to decide which prevention actions to take based on the latest information.

[37] We ran two models—one for the period of time prior to the introduction of COVID-19 vaccines (June 14, 2020, through January 3, 2021) and one for the period of time after introduction of COVID-19 vaccines in nursing homes (January 4, 2021, through January 2, 2022). The first nursing home vaccine clinics were held on December 21, 2020. According to CDC, it takes 2 weeks or more for a vaccine to reach full effectiveness, so we set the start date for the period after the introduction of vaccines as 2 weeks after the first vaccine clinics. See appendix II for a detailed description of our methodology.

[38] Throughout the pandemic there have been changes to federal, state, and local COVID- 19 policies, improvements in infection prevention and control practices, increased availability of personal protective equipment, and improvements to and increased availability for COVID-19 testing. We have previously reported on the importance of infection prevention and control practices and CDC continues to emphasize the importance of rigorous infection prevention and control practices to prevent the spread of COVID-19 in nursing homes. See GAO-22-105133.

outbreaks were shorter—when compared to nursing homes in counties with high community spread.

The magnitude of the association of community spread on outbreak duration was particularly pronounced prior to the introduction of vaccines. Specifically, in the period of time prior to the introduction of vaccines, our model estimated that the duration of a COVID-19 outbreak in a nursing home located in a county experiencing low community spread was approximately 7 days shorter than homes located in counties experiencing high community spread. Even after the introduction of COVID-19 vaccines, community spread was still associated with outbreak duration—the outbreak duration was an estimated 5 days shorter for homes located in counties experiencing low community spread compared to homes located in counties experiencing high community spread.

The number of ongoing outbreaks in a given week throughout the period of review was typically much lower in nursing homes located in counties experiencing low community spread compared to nursing homes located in counties experiencing high community spread. These results could indicate that, during times of higher levels of community spread, staff have a greater likelihood of being exposed to the virus in the community and then bringing it into the nursing home.[39] As we previously noted, the first week of most outbreaks (about 75 percent) coincided with a reported staff case rather than a reported resident case. The importance of community spread in determining the probability of an outbreak ending is consistent with what we found in our literature review, with many studies finding that community spread was associated with the presence and severity of COVID-19 within a nursing home.[40]

---

[39] We recognize that staff may live or visit counties outside of the one where the nursing home is located, but there are no data available to determine this. In addition, visitors, when allowed, could also bring COVID-19 into the nursing home, but there are no data available on nursing home visitors.

[40] For example, one study found that the prevalence of COVID-19 in the community was the strongest predictor of COVID-19 cases and deaths in nursing homes. See Rebecca J. Gorges and R. Tamara Konetzka, "Staffing Levels and COVID-19 Cases and Outbreaks in U.S. Nursing Homes," *Journal of the American Geriatrics Society*, vol. 68, no. 11 (2020): 2462-2466. Another study found that county-level COVID-19 rates and per-capita income were the most significant predictors of COVID-19 outbreaks within nursing homes. See Margaret M. Sugg et al., "Mapping community-level determinants of COVID-19 transmission in nursing homes: A multi-scale approach," *Science of the Total Environment*, vol. 752 (2021). And a third study identified a nursing home's county infection rate as one of the strongest predictors of COVID-19 infection. See Christopher L.F. Sun et al., "Predicting Coronavirus Disease 2019 Infection Risk and Related Risk Drivers in Nursing Homes: A Machine Learning Approach," *JAMDA*, vol. 21, no. 11 (2020): 1533-1538.

Nursing Home Size

The size of a nursing home, as measured by the number of Medicare- or Medicaid-certified beds, was also strongly associated with the duration of a COVID-19 outbreak in a nursing home throughout our period of review. Specifically, we found that small (fewer than 50 beds) and medium (50 to 99 beds) nursing homes had a higher probability of their outbreaks ending during a given week—meaning their outbreaks were shorter—when compared to large (100 to 199 beds) and very large (200 or more beds) nursing homes.

The association of nursing home size with outbreak duration remained fairly consistent both before and after the introduction of vaccines. Specifically, in the period of time prior to the introduction of vaccines, our model estimated that the duration of a COVID-19 outbreak in a small nursing home was just over 2.5 days shorter than large and very large homes and, after the introduction of vaccines, the association decreased slightly to just under an estimated 2.5 days shorter.

These findings may be a result of smaller homes simply having fewer residents and staff who can get infected by the virus, so the outbreaks do not continue for as long as in larger nursing homes. However, it could also be affected by other differences between smaller and larger nursing homes, such as fewer staff and visitors entering smaller nursing homes, which could decrease the likelihood of continued transmission of the virus. The importance of nursing home size being associated with the probability of an outbreak ending is consistent with what we found in our literature review, with multiple studies finding that larger homes were associated with the presence of COVID-19 or higher numbers of COVID- 19 cases.[41]

Staff Shortages

Nursing home-reported staff shortages were also strongly associated with the duration of COVID-19 outbreaks prior to the introduction of vaccines. We

---

[41] For example, one study found that, as of May 2020, larger nursing home size was significantly associated with both an increased probability of having a COVID-19 case and having a larger outbreak. See Hannah R. Abrams et al., "Characteristics of U.S. Nursing Homes with COVID-19 Cases," *Journal of the American Geriatrics Society*, vol. 68, no. 8 (2020): 1653-1656. Another study found that, from March to August 2020, large nursing homes (150 or more beds) reported 2.6 fewer staff COVID-19 cases per 100 beds compared with small nursing homes (less than 50 beds). See Kira L. Ryskina et al., "Characteristics of Nursing Homes by COVID-19 Cases among Staff: March to August 2020," *JAMDA*, vol. 22, no. 5 (2021): 960-965.

found that nursing homes that reported staff shortages had a lower probability of their outbreaks ending during a given week—meaning their outbreaks were longer—when compared to homes that did not report staff shortages.[42]

Prior to the introduction of vaccines, the magnitude of the association of reported staff shortages on outbreak duration was substantial, but the association was minimal after the introduction of vaccines. Specifically, our model estimated that, prior to the introduction of vaccines, the duration of an outbreak at a nursing home reporting staff shortages was over a day longer than homes that did not report shortages. After the introduction of vaccines, the magnitude of the association of nursing home-reported staff shortages on outbreak duration decreased to less than half a day.

These findings may be due to the associated effects of staff shortages. For instance, nurse staff may need to cover more residents and rooms or temporary staff from other homes or health care settings may need to fill the vacancies, both of which could inadvertently cause the virus to be brought into the home or spread throughout more of the home. As previously noted, nursing homes, state survey agencies, and state long- term care ombudsmen we interviewed described staff shortages and associated challenges, such as adhering to CDC-recommended infection prevention and control practices, as concerns during the pandemic.

We also analyzed variables that directly measure actual nursing home staff levels, rather than perceived shortages reported by nursing home officials, and found less clear results. For instance, prior to the introduction of vaccines, the greater the percentage of new employees, the longer an outbreak lasted, but, while statistically significant, the magnitude of the association was small. After the introduction of vaccines, we found the inverse association—the greater the percentage of new employees, the shorter an outbreak lasted—and, again, the magnitude of the association was statistically significant but small. In addition, we found that the associations of other staffing variables, such as average hours per employee per week and number of employees per resident, on outbreak duration were not always statistically significant.

---

[42] A few studies analyzed the association of various factors with the likelihood of nursing homes reporting staff shortages. For example, two studies found that in mid-2020 reported shortages were greater in nursing homes with COVID-19 cases among residents and staff, as well as in homes with lower quality scores and those serving more Medicaid beneficiaries. See Diane M. Gibson and Jessica Greene, "State Actions and Shortages of Personal Protective Equipment and Staff in U.S. Nursing Homes," *Journal of the American Geriatrics Society*, vol. 68, no. 12 (2020): 2721-2726; and Brian E. McGarry et al., "Severe Staffing and Personal Protective Equipment Shortages Faced By Nursing Homes During the COVID-19 Pandemic," *Health Affairs*, vol. 39, no. 10 (2020): 1812-1821.

Our literature review identified one study that analyzed a measure of outbreaks over time and it found an inverse association with nurse staffing ratings.[43] However, our nuanced results are consistent with other studies in our literature review. For example, one study found that, whereas higher staffing levels increase the probability of having at least one COVID-19 case, higher nurse aide and total nursing hours were associated with a lower probability of a larger outbreak and fewer deaths.[44] Another study found that the average number of unique staff members working in a facility on a given day was strongly associated with COVID-19 outcomes in nursing homes, but that, after staff size was controlled for, there was no clear relationship between COVID-19 outcomes and more traditional measures of staffing.[45]

Ownership

The type of nursing home ownership—whether the home is for-profit, non-profit, or government-owned—was also strongly associated with COVID-19 outbreak duration at times during our period of review. We found that nursing homes designated as non-profit or government-owned had a lower probability of their outbreaks ending during a given week— meaning their outbreaks were longer—when compared to homes designated as for-profit. For instance, our model estimated that the duration of an outbreak in a government-owned nursing home was about 1.5 days longer than in for-profit homes after the introduction of vaccines.

The studies in our literature review that found an association between COVID-19 outcomes in nursing homes and nursing home ownership generally found that non-profit homes did better than for-profit homes on the presence or severity of cases and the number of deaths. For example, one study of California nursing homes found that as of May 1, 2020, the size of COVID-

[43] The study examined the total number of weeks a nursing home was in the top decile of the national distribution of weekly confirmed resident COVID-19 incidence and found that nursing homes with lower nurse staffing ratings had 18 to 22 percent more weeks with high COVID-19 incidence than homes with the highest staffing rating. See Christianna S. Williams et al., "The Association of Nursing Home Quality Ratings and Spread of COVID- 19," *Journal of the American Geriatrics Society*, vol. 69, no. 8 (2021): 2070-2078.

[44] See Rebecca J. Gorges and R. Tamara Konetzka, "Staffing Levels and COVID-19 Cases and Outbreaks in U.S. Nursing Homes," *Journal of the American Geriatrics Society*, vol. 68, no. 11 (2020): 2462-2466.

[45] See Brian E. McGarry et al., "Larger Nursing Home Staff Size Linked To Higher Number Of COVID-19 Case In 2020," *Health Affairs*, vol. 40, no. 8 (2021): 1261-1269.

19 outbreaks was 12.7 times larger in for-profit nursing homes than in their non-profit counterparts.[46] One study, however, found an inverse association—that, between March and August 2020, for-profit nursing homes were associated with fewer staff COVID-19 cases when compared to non-profit homes. While our results were unexpected based on the general findings of the studies we reviewed, we analyzed a longer period of time and measured a different outcome— outbreak duration rather than the presence or severity of COVID-19 cases or deaths.

List of Addressees

The Honorable Patrick Leahy
Chairman

The Honorable Richard Shelby
Vice Chairman
Committee on Appropriations
United States Senate

The Honorable Ron Wyden
Chairman
The Honorable Mike Crapo
Ranking Member
Committee on Finance
United States Senate

The Honorable Patty Murray
Chairman

The Honorable Richard Burr
Ranking Member
Committee on Health, Education, Labor, and Pensions
United States Senate

---

[46] See Ram Gopal, Xu Han, and Niam Yaraghi, "Compress the Curve: A Cross-Sectional Study of Variations in COVID-19 Infections across California Nursing Homes," *BMJ Open*, vol. 11 (2021): e042804.

The Honorable Gary C. Peters
Chairman

The Honorable Rob Portman
Ranking Member
Committee on Homeland Security and Governmental Affairs
United States Senate

The Honorable Rosa L. DeLauro
Chair

The Honorable Kay Granger
Ranking Member
Committee on Appropriations
House of Representatives

The Honorable Frank Pallone, Jr.
Chairman

The Honorable Cathy McMorris Rodgers
Republican Leader
Committee on Energy and Commerce
House of Representatives

The Honorable Bennie G. Thompson
Chairman
The Honorable John Katko
Ranking Member
Committee on Homeland Security
House of Representatives

The Honorable Carolyn B. Maloney
Chairwoman

The Honorable James Comer
Ranking Member
Committee on Oversight and Reform
House of Representatives

The Honorable Richard E. Neal
Chair

The Honorable Kevin Brady
Republican Leader
Committee on Ways and Means
House of Representatives

The Honorable Michael F. Bennet
United States Senate

Appendix I: Literature Review—Methodology Description and Results

To understand what is known about the factors associated with COVID- 19 outbreaks in nursing homes, we conducted a systematic literature review from January 1, 2020, through October 1, 2021.

Methodology

We conducted a systematic literature review of studies using data to examine the association of any factor with COVID-19 outbreaks in U.S. nursing homes. We searched across five research platforms (EBSCO, Scopus, SSRN, ProQuest, and Dialog's 96 databases), focusing on those databases that covered health and medical issues.[47] We conducted additional targeted internet searches using the Harvard Kennedy School Think Tank Search to capture additional studies. After reviewing the initial returns from our search, we expanded and updated our search strategy to increase the relevance and breadth of our returns. We ultimately searched the original five research platforms plus PubMed and Google Scholar, covering the time period of January 1, 2020, through October 1, 2021.

We identified a total of 49 studies that met our selection criteria, and we conducted a high-level quality review to assess the reliability and methodological soundness of those studies. We considered studies to be

[47] For instance, Embase, EMCare, HSELINE: Health and Safety, Global Health, Medline, and the New England Journal of Medicine.

sufficiently reliable if they had been peer-reviewed and published in an academic journal, if they were included in a federal or state government publication with similarly rigorous review processes, or if they were prepared by or on behalf of a federal or state government entity.[48] As a result of this process, we determined that 43 studies were sufficiently reliable for our use. We excluded three of those studies because, upon further review, they did not meet our original criteria—to select studies that examined the association of one or more factors with COVID-19 outbreaks in U.S. nursing homes. This resulted in a total of 40 selected studies.

To review these selected studies, we applied a framework of three analytical categories describing the type of analysis conducted for each study: presence, severity, and duration of COVID-19 outbreaks in nursing homes. Some studies conducted more than one of these types of analyses.

- *Presence of COVID-19 outbreaks.* Studies investigating the presence of COVID-19 outbreaks assessed the association of state, county, nursing home, or resident factors with a categorical or binary outcome relating to whether or not COVID-19 affected a nursing home. For example, some studies compared nursing homes that had at least one COVID-19 case or death with homes that did not have any COVID-19 cases or deaths. Eighteen studies were categorized as assessing presence.
- *Severity of COVID-19 outbreaks.* Studies investigating the severity of COVID-19 outbreaks assessed the association of state, county, nursing home, or resident factors with a continuous outcome, such as by comparing the cumulative number of COVID-19 cases or deaths in each nursing home. Thirty-three studies were categorized as assessing severity.

---

[48] If studies did not meet this criterion, we considered them to be sufficiently reliable if they met all of the following three criteria: (1) the study was marked as provisional (e.g., pre-publication status) for a peer-reviewed journal or government publication with a similarly rigorous review process; (2) the study was transparent about its data sources and methods, those sources and methods appeared appropriate for the researchable questions, and the study discussed possible limitations; and (3) the study reported all relevant results, and conclusions and recommendations were adequately supported by those results.
Due to the rapidly evolving nature of the COVID-19 pandemic, we recognized that recent studies may not have had time to complete the full peer review process. We chose to include studies still pending peer review because they could cover emerging issues or use more timely and complete data than studies from earlier in the pandemic. Four of the final 40 studies were marked as provisional at the time of selection. All four of those studies were published by the time of our reporting—three in peer reviewed journals.

Table 2. Studies included in GAO's review that focused on factors associated with the presence, severity, or duration of COVID-19 outbreaks in nursing homes, January 1, 2020, through October 1, 2021

			Methodological focus of study			
	Title	Authors Journal Publication date	Factors associated with the presence of COVID-19 outbreaks in nursing homes	Factors associated with the severity of COVID-19 outbreaks in nursing homes	Factors associated with the duration of COVID-19 outbreaks in nursing homes	Summary of key findings
1	"Is There a Link between Nursing Home Reported Quality and COVID-19 Cases? Evidence from California Skilled Nursing Facilities"	He, Mengying, Yumeng Li, and Fang Fang *JAMDA* July 2020	√	√	–	In California from April 23, 2020, through June 2, 2020, nursing homes with a five-star rating and a higher percentage of White residents were less likely to have COVID-19 cases and deaths compared to other nursing homes in the state, after adjusting for nursing home size, ownership, and years of operation.
2	"Nursing Home Characteristics Associated with COVID-19 Deaths in Connecticut, New Jersey, and New York"	Unruh, Mark Aaron et al. *JAMDA* July 2020	√	–	–	As of mid-April 2020, nursing homes in Connecticut, New Jersey, and New York with the highest percentages of Medicaid patients had an 8.6 percentage point greater probability of six or more COVID-19 deaths than nursing homes with the lowest percentages of these patients in the same three states.

Table 2. (Continued)

			Methodological focus of study			
	Title	Authors Journal Publication date	Factors associated with the presence of COVID-19 outbreaks in nursing homes	Factors associated with the severity of COVID-19 outbreaks in nursing homes	Factors associated with the duration of COVID-19 outbreaks in nursing homes	Summary of key findings
						Other characteristics associated with COVID-19 deaths included having patients with higher activities of daily living scores, more total beds, higher occupancy rates, and being for-profit.
3	"Nurse Staffing and Coronavirus Infections in California Nursing Homes"	Harrington, Charlene et al. *Policy, Politics, & Nursing Practice* July 7, 2020	√	–	–	Between March and May 2020, California nursing homes with total registered nurse staffing levels under 0.75 hours per resident day had a two times greater probability of having COVID-19 resident infections. Nursing homes with lower Medicare five-star ratings on total nurse and registered nurse staffing levels (adjusted for acuity), higher total health deficiencies, and more beds had a higher probability of having COVID-19 residents.

			Methodological focus of study			
	Title	Authors Journal Publication date	Factors associated with the presence of COVID-19 outbreaks in nursing homes	Factors associated with the severity of COVID-19 outbreaks in nursing homes	Factors associated with the duration of COVID-19 outbreaks in nursing homes	Summary of key findings
4	"Characteristics and Quality of US Nursing Homes Reporting Cases of Coronavirus Disease 2019 (COVID-19)"	Chatterjee, Paula et al. *JAMA Network Open* July 29, 2020	√	–	–	In nursing homes from the District of Columbia and 23 states reporting COVID-19 cases from April 22, 2020, through April, 29, 2020, homes that reported COVID-19 cases had similar mean scores as those that did not on overall five-star ratings, as well as star ratings on deficiencies and staffing. Compared to homes that did not report cases, those that did had higher rates of health deficiencies, emergency preparedness deficiencies, reported incidents, and substantiated complaints. Rates of COVID-19 were nearly twice as high in counties where homes reported COVID-19 cases than in those without reported cases.

Table 2. (Continued)

			Methodological focus of study			
	Title	Authors Journal Publication date	Factors associated with the presence of COVID-19 outbreaks in nursing homes	Factors associated with the severity of COVID-19 outbreaks in nursing homes	Factors associated with the duration of COVID-19 outbreaks in nursing homes	Summary of key findings
5	"Characteristics of U.S. Nursing Homes with COVID-19 Cases"	Abrams, Hannah R. et al. *Journal of the American Geriatrics Society* August 2020	√	√	–	In all nursing homes from 30 states with facility-level COVID-19 data as of May 11, 2020, larger facility size, urban location, greater percentage of African American residents, non-chain status, and state were significantly related to the increased probability of having a COVID-19 case. Five- star rating, prior infection violation, Medicaid dependency, and ownership were not significantly related. The size of the outbreak was significantly associated with facility size, for-profit status, and state but not with other studied characteristics.

			Methodological focus of study			
	Title	Authors Journal Publication date	Factors associated with the presence of COVID-19 outbreaks in nursing homes	Factors associated with the severity of COVID-19 outbreaks in nursing homes	Factors associated with the duration of COVID-19 outbreaks in nursing homes	Summary of key findings
6	"Mapping Community-Level Determinants of COVID-19 Transmission in Nursing homes: A Multi-Scale Approach"	Sugg, Margaret M. et al. *Science of the Total Environment* August 25, 2020	√	√	–	As of June 30, 2020, county-level COVID-19 rates, per-capita income, average household size, population density, unemployment, and a higher percentage of African Americans, in combination with nursing home staffing levels (licensed practical nurses and total staff) and number of fines issued in 2020 were associated with an increased risk of COVID-19 cases in nursing homes. Lower overall quality rating and staffing rating increased the risk of COVID-19 cases, but the results were not statistically significant
7	"Staffing Levels and COVID-19 Cases and Outbreaks in U.S. Nursing Homes"	Gorges, Rebecca J. and R. Tamara Konetzka Journal of the American Geriatrics Society August 28, 2020	√	√	–	As of June 14, 2020, higher registered nurse-hours were associated with a higher probability of a nursing home experiencing any COVID-19 cases. However, among nursing homes with at least one case, higher nurse aide hours and total nursing hours were associated with a lower probability of

Table 2. (Continued)

			Methodological focus of study			
	Title	Authors Journal Publication date	Factors associated with the presence of COVID-19 outbreaks in nursing homes	Factors associated with the severity of COVID-19 outbreaks in nursing homes	Factors associated with the duration of COVID-19 outbreaks in nursing homes	Summary of key findings
						experiencing an outbreak and with fewer deaths. The strongest predictor of cases and outbreaks in nursing homes was per capita cases in the county.
8	"COVID-19 Infections and Deaths among Connecticut Nursing Home Residents: Facility Correlates"	Li, Yue et al. *Journal of the American Geriatrics Society* September 2020	√	√	–	Among Connecticut nursing homes with at least one confirmed COVID-19 case, as of April 16, 2020, every 20-minute increase in registered nurse staffing (per resident day) was associated with 22 percent fewer confirmed cases. Compared with one- to three-star facilities, four- or five-star facilities had 13 percent fewer confirmed cases, and facilities with a high concentration of Medicaid residents or racial/ethnic minority residents had 16 percent and 15 percent more confirmed cases, respectively, than their counterparts. Among nursing

			Methodological focus of study			
	Title	Authors Journal Publication date	Factors associated with the presence of COVID-19 outbreaks in nursing homes	Factors associated with the severity of COVID-19 outbreaks in nursing homes	Factors associated with the duration of COVID-19 outbreaks in nursing homes	Summary of key findings
						homes with at least one COVID-19 death, every 20- minute increase in registered nurse staffing significantly predicted 26 percent fewer COVID-19 deaths. Other characteristics did not show statistically significant associations with COVID-19 deaths.
9	"Association of Nursing Home Ratings on Health Inspections, Quality of Care, and Nurse Staffing with COVID- 19 Cases"	Figueroa, Jose F. et al. *JAMA* September 15, 2020	–	√	–	For 4,254 nursing homes across eight states from January 1, 2020, through June 30, 2020, nursing homes with high ratings on nurse staffing had fewer COVID-19 cases than nursing homes with low ratings on nurse staffing. There was no significant association between high- and low-performing nursing homes in the health inspections or quality measures domains with COVID-19 cases.

Table 2. (Continued)

			Methodological focus of study			
	Title	Authors Journal Publication date	Factors associated with the presence of COVID-19 outbreaks in nursing homes	Factors associated with the severity of COVID-19 outbreaks in nursing homes	Factors associated with the duration of COVID-19 outbreaks in nursing homes	Summary of key findings
10	"Association Between CMS Quality Ratings and COVID-19 Outbreaks in Nursing Homes—West Virginia, March 17-June 11, 2020"	Bui, David P. et al. *Morbidity and Mortality Weekly Report* September 18, 2020	√	–	–	During March through June 2020, 14 (11 percent) of 123 West Virginia nursing homes experienced COVID-19 outbreaks. Compared with one-star–rated (lowest rating) nursing homes, the odds of a COVID- 19 outbreak were 87 percent lower among two- to three-star–rated facilities and 94 percent lower among four- to five-star–rated facilities.
11	"A Study of the COVID-19 Outbreak and Response in Connecticut Long- Term Care Facilities"	Rowan, Patricia et al. *Connecticut Department of Public Health* September 30, 2020	–	√	–	Through July 22, 2020, nursing homes in Connecticut with a high staffing rating had significantly fewer COVID-19 cases and deaths per licensed bed than nursing homes with a lower staffing rating. Nursing homes in Connecticut located in communities with a greater incidence of COVID-19 were more likely to experience higher numbers of cases and deaths. Nursing

			Methodological focus of study			
	Title	Authors Journal Publication date	Factors associated with the presence of COVID-19 outbreaks in nursing homes	Factors associated with the severity of COVID-19 outbreaks in nursing homes	Factors associated with the duration of COVID-19 outbreaks in nursing homes	Summary of key findings
						homes in Connecticut with a larger share of residents that received dialysis and cancer treatments, which tend to be delivered off site, had more cases per licensed bed. The total number of residents and the share of the licensed beds that were filled also significantly predicted greater COVID-19 spread.
12	"Variation in SARS- CoV-2 Prevalence in U.S. Skilled Nursing Facilities"	White, Elizabeth M. et al. *Journal of the American Geriatrics Society* October 2020	√	√	–	As of late April and early May 2020, a difference in county prevalence of 1,000 COVID-19 cases per 100,000 (1 percent) was associated with a 33.6 percentage point difference in the probability of an outbreak for Genesis HealthCare-owned nursing homes (sample of 341 nursing homes in 25 states) and non-Genesis nursing homes (sample of 3,016 nursing homes in 12 states) combined, and a difference of 12.5 cases per facility for Genesis nursing homes. A 10-bed difference in facility size was associated with a 0.9

Table 2. (Continued)

			Methodological focus of study			
	Title	Authors Journal Publication date	Factors associated with the presence of COVID-19 outbreaks in nursing homes	Factors associated with the severity of COVID-19 outbreaks in nursing homes	Factors associated with the duration of COVID-19 outbreaks in nursing homes	Summary of key findings
						percentage point difference in the probability of outbreak. No consistent relationship was found between nursing home Five-Star ratings or past infection control deficiency citations and probability or severity of outbreak.
13	"Prevalence of COVID-19 in Ohio Nursing Homes: What's Quality Got to Do with It?"	Bowblis, John and Robert Applebaum *Journal of Aging & Social Policy* October 11, 2020	√	√	–	Through mid-June 2020, just under one-third of nursing homes in Ohio had at least one resident with COVID-19, with over 82 percent of all cases in the state coming from 37 percent of nursing homes. Overall findings on the association between facility quality and the prevalence of COVID-19 showed that having any resident case of the virus or even having a high caseload of residents with the virus is not more likely in nursing homes with lower quality ratings.

			Methodological focus of study			
	Title	Authors Journal Publication date	Factors associated with the presence of COVID-19 outbreaks in nursing homes	Factors associated with the severity of COVID-19 outbreaks in nursing homes	Factors associated with the duration of COVID-19 outbreaks in nursing homes	Summary of key findings
14	"Comparative Performance of Private Equity- Owned US Nursing Homes During the COVID-19 pandemic	Braun, Robert Tyler et al. *JAMA Network Open* October 28, 2020	–	√	–	From May 17, 2020, through July 2, 2020, there were no statistically significant differences in staffing levels, COVID-19 cases or deaths, or deaths by any cause between private equity-owned nursing homes and for-profit, nonprofit, and government-owned facilities. For-profit, nonprofit, and government-owned nursing homes were more likely to have at least a 1-week supply of N95 masks and a 1-week supply of medical gowns than private equity- owned nursing homes.
15	"Mortality Rates from COVID-19 Are Lower in Unionized Nursing Homes"	Dean, Adam, Atheendar Venkataramani, and Simeon Kimmel Health Affairs November 2020	–	√	–	In 355 New York nursing homes with available data from March 1, 2020, through May 31, 2020, health care worker unions were associated with a 1.29 percentage point decrease in the COVID-19 mortality when compared

Table 2. (Continued)

			Methodological focus of study			
	Title	Authors Journal Publication date	Factors associated with the presence of COVID-19 outbreaks in nursing homes	Factors associated with the severity of COVID-19 outbreaks in nursing homes	Factors associated with the duration of COVID-19 outbreaks in nursing homes	Summary of key findings
						with nursing homes without these unions. Unions were also associated with greater access to personal protective equipment.
16	"Racial and Ethnic Disparities in COVID- 19 Infections and Deaths Across U.S. Nursing Homes"	Li, Yue et al. *Journal of the American Geriatrics Society* November 2020	√	√	–	For COVID-19 data reported the week of May 25, 2020, nursing homes with a high- proportion of racial and ethnic minorities were 76 percent more likely to have at least one new resident case compared to nursing homes with a low-proportion of racial and ethnic minorities. In addition, similar across-facility disparities were found for the weekly count of new COVID-19 deaths among residents and in the weekly count of new COVID-19 confirmed cases among staff. No substantial disparities in self-reported shortages of staff or personal protective equipment were found.

			Methodological focus of study			
	Title	Authors Journal Publication date	Factors associated with the presence of COVID-19 outbreaks in nursing homes	Factors associated with the severity of COVID-19 outbreaks in nursing homes	Factors associated with the duration of COVID-19 outbreaks in nursing homes	Summary of key findings
17	"Stemming the Tide of COVID-19 Infections in Massachusetts Nursing Homes"	Lipsitz, Lewis A. et al. *Journal of the American Geriatrics Society* November 2020	–	√	–	In response to the COVID-19 pandemic, a statewide effort in Massachusetts offered all 360 nursing homes in the state weekly webinars and answers to questions regarding infection control procedures. The effort also targeted a subset of 123 nursing homes with previous infection control deficiencies for intervention, which included on-site and virtual consultations. During the 9-week intervention period from May 10, 2020, through July 5, 2020, both resident and staff COVID-19 infection rates started higher in the targeted subset of nursing homes, then rapidly declined to the same low level as other nursing homes.

Table 2. (Continued)

			Methodological focus of study			
	Title	Authors Journal Publication date	Factors associated with the presence of COVID-19 outbreaks in nursing homes	Factors associated with the severity of COVID-19 outbreaks in nursing homes	Factors associated with the duration of COVID-19 outbreaks in nursing homes	Summary of key findings
						Adherence to infection control processes, especially proper wearing of personal protective equipment and cohorting, was significantly associated with declines in weekly infection and mortality rates.
18	"Predicting Coronavirus Disease 2019 Infection Risk and Related Risk Drivers in Nursing Homes: A Machine Learning Approach"	Sun, Christopher L.F. et al. *JAMDA* November 2020	√	–	–	As of April 20, 2020, the strongest predictors of COVID-19 cases in 1,146 nursing homes in Massachusetts, Georgia, and New Jersey were the nursing home's county's infection rate and the number of separate units in the nursing home; other predictors included the county's population density, the nursing home's historical health deficiency citations, and the nursing home's resident density (in persons per 1,000 square feet). In addition, the nursing home's historical percentage of non-Hispanic White

			Methodological focus of study			
	Title	Authors Journal Publication date	Factors associated with the presence of COVID-19 outbreaks in nursing homes	Factors associated with the severity of COVID-19 outbreaks in nursing homes	Factors associated with the duration of COVID-19 outbreaks in nursing homes	Summary of key findings
						residents was identified as a protective factor.
19	"The Role of the Social Vulnerability Index in Personal Protective Equipment Shortages, Number of Cases, and Associated Mortality During the Coronavirus Disease 2019 (COVID-19) Pandemic in Michigan Skilled Nursing Facilities"	LeRose, Jennifer J. et al. *Infection Control & Hospital Epidemiology* November 13, 2020	–	√	–	In May 2020, Michigan nursing homes located in the most vulnerable areas of the state, which was determined using the Centers for Disease Control and Prevention's social vulnerability index, were 2.3 times more likely to experience personal protective equipment shortages than homes located in the least vulnerable areas. In addition, nursing homes located in the most vulnerable areas had 1.6 times the number of COVID-19 cases and 1.9 times the mortality rate compared to nursing homes located in the least vulnerable areas.

Table 2. (Continued)

			Methodological focus of study			
	Title	Authors Journal Publication date	Factors associated with the presence of COVID-19 outbreaks in nursing homes	Factors associated with the severity of COVID-19 outbreaks in nursing homes	Factors associated with the duration of COVID-19 outbreaks in nursing homes	Summary of key findings
20	"Nursing Home Staff Networks and COVID-19"	Chen, M. Keith, Judith A. Chevalier, and Elisa F. Long *Proceedings of the National Academy of Sciences* December 28, 2020	–	√	–	During the 11-week period from March 13, 2020, to May 31, 2020, 5.1 percent of 50 million smartphone users who visited a nursing home for at least one hour also visited another nursing home and nursing homes, on average, shared connections with an estimated 7.1 other homes. Comparing demographically and geographically situated nursing homes of similar quality suggested that 49 percent of nursing home COVID-19 cases were attributable to shared staff transmitting the virus across multiple nursing homes
21	"Compress the Curve: A Cross-Sectional Study of Variations in COVID- 19 Infections across California Nursing Homes"	Gopal, Ram, Xu Han, and Niam Yaraghi *BMJ Open* January 6, 2021	√	√	–	For California nursing homes as of May 1, 2020, the size of COVID-19 outbreaks among residents in for-profit nursing homes was 12.7 times larger than their non-profit counterparts.

			Methodological focus of study			
	Title	Authors Journal Publication date	Factors associated with the presence of COVID-19 outbreaks in nursing homes	Factors associated with the severity of COVID-19 outbreaks in nursing homes	Factors associated with the duration of COVID-19 outbreaks in nursing homes	Summary of key findings
						Higher star ratings for health inspections were associated with a lower number of infections among both staff and residents and higher star ratings for staffing were associated with a lower number of infections among residents. Conversely, higher star ratings for quality measures were associated with a higher number of infections among staff and residents.
22	"Factors Associated with Racial Differences in Deaths Among Nursing Home Residents with COVID-19 Infection in the U.S."	Gorges, Rebecca J. and R. Tamara Konetzka *JAMA Network Open* February 10, 2021	–	√	–	As of September 13, 2020, nursing homes in which more than 40 percent of residents were non-White experienced case and death counts that were 3.3-fold higher than those of nursing homes with low proportions of non-White residents.

Table 2. (Continued)

			Methodological focus of study			
	Title	Authors Journal Publication date	Factors associated with the presence of COVID-19 outbreaks in nursing homes	Factors associated with the severity of COVID-19 outbreaks in nursing homes	Factors associated with the duration of COVID-19 outbreaks in nursing homes	Summary of key findings
						These differences in resident deaths by race were associated with nursing home size and community-level outbreak severity, but not with aggregate health status of residents or other nursing home characteristics.
23	"Nontraditional Small House Nursing Homes Have Fewer COVID-19 Cases and Deaths"	Zimmerman, Sheryl et al. *JAMDA* March 2021	–	√	–	Green House and other small nursing home models are considered nontraditional due to their size (10-12 beds), universal caregivers, and other home-like features. From January 20, 2020, through July 31, 2020, 219 Green House and other similar small nursing homes located in 20 states had lower COVID-19 incidence and mortality rates compared to 392 geographically proximate traditional nursing homes, especially among the higher and extreme values.

			Methodological focus of study			
	Title	Authors Journal Publication date	Factors associated with the presence of COVID-19 outbreaks in nursing homes	Factors associated with the severity of COVID-19 outbreaks in nursing homes	Factors associated with the duration of COVID-19 outbreaks in nursing homes	Summary of key findings
24	"Predicting COVID- 19 at Skilled Nursing Facilities in California: Do the Stars Align?"	Poltavskiy, Eduard et al. *BMJ Open Quality* March 3, 2021	√	–	–	As of May 31, 2020, publicly reported nursing home metrics were associated with COVID-19 presence in California nursing homes. Specifically, nursing home health inspection star ratings, emergency room visits, and short-stay hospitalizations were significantly associated with nursing homes reporting COVID-19 cases.
25	"High-Minority Nursing Homes Disproportionately Affected by COVID- 19 Deaths"	Weech- Maldonado, Robert et al. *Frontiers in Public Health* March 22, 2021	–	√	–	As of October 25, 2020, nursing homes with a high percentage of minority residents reported 6.5 COVID-19 deaths as compared to 2.6 deaths for nursing homes that had no racial or ethnic minorities. After controlling for interstate differences, facility-level resident characteristics, resource availability, and organizational characteristics, nursing homes with a

Table 2. (Continued)

			Methodological focus of study			
	Title	Authors Journal Publication date	Factors associated with the presence of COVID-19 outbreaks in nursing homes	Factors associated with the severity of COVID-19 outbreaks in nursing homes	Factors associated with the duration of COVID-19 outbreaks in nursing homes	Summary of key findings
						high percentage of minority residents had 61 percent more COVID-19 deaths as compared to nursing homes with no minorities.
26	"Assessment of Coronavirus Disease 2019 Infection and Mortality Rates among Nursing Homes with Different Proportions of Black Residents"	Travers, Jasmine L. et al. *JAMDA* April 2021	–	√	–	From January 20, 2020, through July 19, 2020, nursing homes with any Black residents showed significantly more COVID- 19 infections and deaths than nursing homes with no Black residents. There were 13.6 percentage points more infections and 3.5 percentage points more deaths in nursing homes with 50 percent or greater Black residents than in nursing homes with no Black residents. Although facility characteristics explained some of the differences found in multivariable analyses, county-level factors and rurality explained more of the differences.

			Methodological focus of study			
	Title	Authors Journal Publication date	Factors associated with the presence of COVID-19 outbreaks in nursing homes	Factors associated with the severity of COVID-19 outbreaks in nursing homes	Factors associated with the duration of COVID-19 outbreaks in nursing homes	Summary of key findings
27	"Short-Term Impact of Nursing Home SARS-CoV-2 Vaccinations on New Infections, Hospitalizations, and Deaths"	Mor, Vincent et al. *Journal of the American Geriatrics Society* April 16, 2021	–	√	–	Two hundred and eighty nursing homes in 21 states owned and operated by Genesis Healthcare were divided into two COVID-19 vaccination groups based on the date the nursing home had its initial vaccine clinic— early vaccination group (December 18, 2020, through January 2, 2021) and late vaccination group (January 3, 2021, through January 18, 2021). After 1 week, early vaccinated nursing homes had a predicted 2.5 fewer incident COVID-19 infections per 100 at-risk residents per week compared with what would have been expected based on the experience of the late vaccinated nursing homes. The rates remained significantly lower for several weeks.

Table 2. (Continued)

			Methodological focus of study			
	Title	Authors Journal Publication date	Factors associated with the presence of COVID-19 outbreaks in nursing homes	Factors associated with the severity of COVID-19 outbreaks in nursing homes	Factors associated with the duration of COVID-19 outbreaks in nursing homes	Summary of key findings
28	"SARS-CoV-2 in Nursing Homes after 3 Months of Serial, Faciltywide Point Prevalence Testing, Connecticut, USA"	Ehrlich, Hanna Y. et al. *Emerging Infectious Diseases* May 2021	–	√	–	The Connecticut Department of Public Health began point prevalence survey testing in nursing homes in early May 2020, and this type of testing was formally recommended on May 11, 2020, and mandated weekly in staff effective June 14, 2020. The state initially prioritized a subset of 34 Connecticut nursing homes to receive test kits and these nursing homes performed their first round of testing on or before May 20, 2020. After adjusting for community incidence of COVID- 19, the implementation of serial point prevalence survey testing in the 34 nursing homes was associated with a significant decrease in nursing home COVID-19 incidence rates compared to the pre- implementation period.

			Methodological focus of study			
	Title	Authors Journal Publication date	Factors associated with the presence of COVID-19 outbreaks in nursing homes	Factors associated with the severity of COVID-19 outbreaks in nursing homes	Factors associated with the duration of COVID-19 outbreaks in nursing homes	Summary of key findings
29	"Shifting US Patterns of COVID-19 Mortality by Race and Ethnicity from June-December 2020"	Kumar, Amit et al. *JAMDA* May 2021	–	√	–	During the first 6 weeks of a 30-week study period, which started on June 1, 2020, nursing homes with a higher proportion of Black residents reported more COVID-19 deaths per 1,000 followed by nursing homes with a higher proportion of Hispanic residents. Between 7 and 12 weeks, nursing homes with a higher proportion of Hispanic residents reported more deaths per 1,000, followed by nursing homes with a higher proportion of Black residents. However, after 23 weeks (mid-November 2020), nursing homes serving a higher proportion of White residents reported more deaths per 1,000 than nursing homes serving a high proportion of Black and Hispanic residents.

Table 2. (Continued)

			Methodological focus of study			
	Title	Authors Journal Publication date	Factors associated with the presence of COVID-19 outbreaks in nursing homes	Factors associated with the severity of COVID-19 outbreaks in nursing homes	Factors associated with the duration of COVID-19 outbreaks in nursing homes	Summary of key findings
30	"Characteristics of Nursing Homes by COVID-19 Cases Among Staff: March to August 2020"	Ryskina, Kira L. et al. *JAMDA* May 2021	–	√	–	From March to August 2020, after accounting for local COVID-19 prevalence, nursing homes in the highest quartile of confirmed resident cases reported 18.9 more staff cases per 100 beds compared with nursing homes that had no resident cases. Large nursing homes (150 or more beds) reported 2.6 fewer staff cases per 100 beds compared with small nursing homes (<50 beds) and for-profit nursing homes reported 0.8 fewer staff cases per 100 beds compared with nonprofit nursing homes. Higher occupancy and more direct-care hours per day were associated with more staff cases. Estimates associated with resident demographics, payer mix, or regional socioeconomic characteristics were not statistically significant.

			Methodological focus of study			
	Title	Authors Journal Publication date	Factors associated with the presence of COVID-19 outbreaks in nursing homes	Factors associated with the severity of COVID-19 outbreaks in nursing homes	Factors associated with the duration of COVID-19 outbreaks in nursing homes	Summary of key findings
31	"The BNT162b2 Vaccine Is Associated with Lower New COVID- 19 Cases in Nursing Home Residents and Staff"	Domi, Marsida et al *Journal of the American Geriatrics Society* May 6, 2021	–	√	–	Dividing the 2,501 nursing homes from the first 17 states to hold vaccine clinics into three groups—vaccine clinic ending the week of December 27, 2020 (cohort 1), January 3, 2021 (cohort 2), or January 10, 2021 (cohort 3)—found that resident and staff cases trended downward in all three cohorts following the vaccine clinic. Time following the first clinic at 5 and 6 weeks was consistently associated with fewer resident cases, resident deaths, and staff cases. Other factors associated with fewer resident and staff cases included facilities with less than 50 beds and high nurse staffing per resident day. Higher Hispanic non-White resident census was associated with fewer resident cases and deaths.

Table 2. (Continued)

			Methodological focus of study			
	Title	Authors Journal Publication date	Factors associated with the presence of COVID-19 outbreaks in nursing homes	Factors associated with the severity of COVID-19 outbreaks in nursing homes	Factors associated with the duration of COVID-19 outbreaks in nursing homes	Summary of key findings
32	"Trends in COVID-19 Death Rates by Racial Composition of Nursing Homes"	Gilman, Matlin and Mary T. Bassett *Journal of the American Geriatrics Society* May 15, 2021	–	√	–	From May 25, 2020 to April 18, 2021, death rates in nursing homes categorized into the highest and lowest quintiles of White residents varied over time. Specifically, high- White quintile nursing homes initially had a lower death rate than low-White quintile nursing homes. However, by late December 2020, high-White quintile nursing homes had experienced 3 months of higher community spread and its death rate had increased to nearly three times that of low-White quintile nursing homes. Through the first few months of 2021, death rates declined substantially for both groups of nursing homes, but, overall, high-White quintile nursing homes had more total deaths than low-White quintile nursing homes despite having fewer beds and higher star ratings.

			Methodological focus of study			
	Title	Authors Journal Publication date	Factors associated with the presence of COVID-19 outbreaks in nursing homes	Factors associated with the severity of COVID-19 outbreaks in nursing homes	Factors associated with the duration of COVID-19 outbreaks in nursing homes	Summary of key findings
33	"The Association of Nursing Home Quality Ratings and Spread of COVID- 19"	Williams, Christianna S. et al. *Journal of the American Geriatrics Society* May 31, 2021	–	√	√	As of January 10, 2021, higher nursing home quality ratings were associated with COVID- 19 incidence and mortality, as well as with fewer high-incidence weeks, after controlling for local community COVID-19 spread and relevant facility-level factors. For example, nursing homes with a lower overall rating (one- to three-stars) had about 10 percent more weeks with high COVID-19 incidence than the highest (five-star) rated homes, and nursing homes with an overall star rating of one- to three-stars also had about 13 to 16 percent higher incidence and 8 to 10 percent higher cumulative COVID-19 mortality than five-star homes.

Table 2. (Continued)

			Methodological focus of study			
	Title	Authors Journal Publication date	Factors associated with the presence of COVID-19 outbreaks in nursing homes	Factors associated with the severity of COVID-19 outbreaks in nursing homes	Factors associated with the duration of COVID-19 outbreaks in nursing homes	Summary of key findings
						Higher county COVID-19 incidence was also strongly and consistently associated with higher nursing home COVID-19 incidence and mortality, as well as number of high-incidence weeks.
34	"Trends in Racial and Ethnic Disparities in Coronavirus Disease 2019 (COVID-19) Outcomes among Nursing Home Residents"	Li, Yue et al. *Infection Control & Hospital Epidemiology* June 16, 2021	–	√	–	From April 13, 2020, through June 19, 2020, Connecticut nursing homes caring for predominately racial and ethnic minority residents tended to have higher COVID-19 incidence and fatality rates. Specifically, compared to nursing homes with a low proportion of racial and ethnic minority residents, the adjusted COVID-19 incidence rate ratios for the nursing homes with a high proportion of racial and ethnic minority residents were 1.18 in week 1 of the study period and 1.54 in week

			Methodological focus of study			
	Title	Authors Journal Publication date	Factors associated with the presence of COVID-19 outbreaks in nursing homes	Factors associated with the severity of COVID-19 outbreaks in nursing homes	Factors associated with the duration of COVID-19 outbreaks in nursing homes	Summary of key findings
						10, showing a 30 percent relative increase. Adjusted disparities in COVID-19 fatalities similarly increased over time.
35	"COVID-19 Cases and Death in Nursing Homes: The Role of Racial and Ethnic Composition of Facilities and Their Communities"	Cai, Shubing, Di Yan, and Orna Intrator *JAMDA* July 2021	√	–	–	From June 7, 2020, through August 23, 2020, the racial and ethnic composition of nursing homes and their communities were both associated with the likelihood of having COVID-19 cases and death in nursing homes. The racial and ethnic composition of the community played an independent role in the likelihood of COVID-19 cases and death in nursing homes, even after accounting for the COVID-19 infection rate in the community. In addition, the relationship between nursing home characteristics and the probability of COVID-19 cases or death varied with the racial and ethnic composition of the community.

Table 2. (Continued)

			Methodological focus of study			
	Title	Authors Journal Publication date	Factors associated with the presence of COVID-19 outbreaks in nursing homes	Factors associated with the severity of COVID-19 outbreaks in nursing homes	Factors associated with the duration of COVID-19 outbreaks in nursing homes	Summary of key findings
						For example, although an hour increase in registered nurse hours per resident per day was associated with 2.8 percentage point reduction in the probability of COVID-19 cases in nursing homes located in high-minority communities, such relationship was smaller in low-minority communities.
36	"Larger Nursing Home Staff Size Linked to Higher Number of COVID- 19 Cases in 2020"	McGarry, Brian E. et al. *Health Affairs* August 2021	–	√	–	From June 7, 2020, through September 27, 2020, sample nursing homes (7,154 nursing homes without resident COVID-19 cases by the start of the study period) in the lowest quartile of staff size had 6.2 resident cases and 0.9 deaths per 100 beds, compared with 11.9 resident cases and 2.1 deaths per 100 beds among nursing homes in the highest quartile. Staff size, including staff members not involved in resident care, was strongly associated with

			Methodological focus of study			
	Title	Authors Journal Publication date	Factors associated with the presence of COVID-19 outbreaks in nursing homes	Factors associated with the severity of COVID-19 outbreaks in nursing homes	Factors associated with the duration of COVID-19 outbreaks in nursing homes	Summary of key findings
						COVID-19 outcomes, even after nursing home size was accounted for. Staffing quality measures, including direct care staff-to-resident ratios and skill mix, were not significant predictors of COVID-19 cases or deaths.
37	"Interpreting COVID- 19 Deaths among Nursing Home Residents in the US: The Changing Role of Facility Quality Over Time"	Das Gupta, Debasree et al. *PLOS ONE* September 1, 2021	√	√	–	From June 1, 2020, through January 31, 2021, nursing homes with a higher overall quality rating were associated with lower rates of COVID-19 deaths. However, this association diminished over the study period. In addition, the duration of self-reported staff shortages by nursing homes were associated with COVID-19 mortality rates and the adverse role of staff shortages did not change over the study period. Nursing home ownership and shortage of personal protective equipment were not associated with COVID-19 mortality at any point during the study period,

Table 2. (Continued)

			Methodological focus of study			
	Title	Authors Journal Publication date	Factors associated with the presence of COVID-19 outbreaks in nursing homes	Factors associated with the severity of COVID-19 outbreaks in nursing homes	Factors associated with the duration of COVID-19 outbreaks in nursing homes	Summary of key findings
						but community level variables (such as local COVID-19 death rate) were significant determinants of nursing home mortality outcomes.
38	"State Social Distancing Restrictions and Nursing Home Outcomes"	Li, Yue et al. *Scientific Reports* January 20, 2022	√	√	–	From June to August 2020, stronger state social distancing measures were associated with lower weekly rates of new COVID-19 confirmed cases and related deaths among nursing home residents, as well as lower weekly COVID-19 new confirmed case rate among nursing home staff. The magnitude of these associations was larger for nursing homes serving disproportionately more racial and ethnic minority residents.

			Methodological focus of study			
	Title	Authors Journal Publication date	Factors associated with the presence of COVID-19 outbreaks in nursing homes	Factors associated with the severity of COVID-19 outbreaks in nursing homes	Factors associated with the duration of COVID-19 outbreaks in nursing homes	Summary of key findings
39	"Nursing Home Quality, COVID-19 Deaths, and Excess Mortality"	Cronin, Christopher J. and William N. Evans *Journal of Health Economics* January 21, 2022	–	√	–	From the start of the pandemic through September 13, 2020, a nursing home's overall five-star rating was highly predictive of COVID-19 mortality, with five-star nursing homes having 15 percent fewer resident COVID-19 deaths than one-star nursing homes. This relationship between quality and COVID-19 deaths did not continue after September 13, 2020, through April 25, 2021. Conversely, higher-quality nursing homes had much higher non-COVID-19 mortality, with five-star nursing homes experiencing 11.4 percent more non-COVID-19 deaths than one-star homes as of September 13, 2020. This relationship strengthened over time through April 2021.

Table 2. (Continued)

			Methodological focus of study			
	Title	Authors Journal Publication date	Factors associated with the presence of COVID-19 outbreaks in nursing homes	Factors associated with the severity of COVID-19 outbreaks in nursing homes	Factors associated with the duration of COVID-19 outbreaks in nursing homes	Summary of key findings
40	"Firm Finances and the Spread of COVID-19: Evidence from Nursing Homes"	Begley, Taylor A., and Daniel Weagley *SSRN* July 28, 2022	–	√	–	For a sample of 7,045 nursing homes, as of October 18, 2020, those nursing homes with less liquidity and those experiencing more severe cash flow shocks had more cases of COVID-19. For example, increased Medicaid nursing home reimbursement rates was associated with much lower rates of COVID- 19 and the difference was largest for nursing homes with the highest share of Medicaid residents.

Notes: We selected studies for inclusion in our review if they used data to examine the association of any factor with COVID-19 outbreaks in U.S. nursing homes. Studies listed in the table used nationwide data except where specific states are indicated in the summary.

- *Duration of COVID-19 outbreaks.* Studies investigating the duration of COVID-19 outbreaks assessed the association of state, county, nursing home, or resident factors with the amount of time that each nursing home was experiencing COVID-19 outbreaks. One study was categorized as assessing duration.

Results

Table 2 lists the 40 studies we reviewed.

Appendix II: Detailed Description of Methodology for Multivariate Statistical Models

This appendix describes our methods for analyzing how certain nursing home factors were associated with the duration of COVID-19 outbreaks. To do this, we used Centers for Disease Control and Prevention (CDC), Centers for Medicare & Medicaid Services (CMS), and Health Resources and Services Administration data to develop Cox proportional hazard statistical models, which simultaneously evaluate the association between many factors on the probability of a specified outcome and the significance of the relationship. Specifically, our models estimated the probability of an outbreak ending at any given week from June 14, 2020, through January 2, 2022, controlling for a host of factors, such as nursing home characteristics and levels of COVID-19 in the surrounding community, among others. The following describes our definitions, data sources, and methodology.

CDC COVID-19 Nursing Home Data

We used CDC's COVID-19 nursing home data as the foundation for our statistical model. CDC collects weekly nursing home-level COVID-19 information, including cases, deaths, and shortages of staff and supplies, from all Medicare- or Medicaid-certified nursing homes.[49] We analyzed the data for

[49] The CDC data on COVID-19 in nursing homes were accessed on May 12, 2022, for the week ending May 1, 2022, from https://data.cms.gov/covid-19/covid-19-nursing-home- data. Nursing homes report aggregate data to CDC on a weekly basis. According to CDC, data used

the week ending June 14, 2020, through the week ending January 2, 2022, the last full week of the 2021 calendar year. CMS began requiring nursing homes to report COVID-19 data to CDC in May 2020. Reporting information retroactively to the beginning of the pandemic was voluntary and the data do not clearly distinguish between nursing homes that opted to report information prior to this time and those that did not. Therefore, we started our analysis with data for the week ending June 14, 2020, and excluded data from the first 3 weeks of reporting because these data contained information from multiple weeks dating back to February 2020.

COVID-19 Outbreaks in Nursing Homes

According to CDC, a COVID-19 outbreak starts the week a nursing home reports a new COVID-19 case in a resident or staff member and ends when the nursing home has 2 consecutive weeks (not included in the outbreak duration) where they report no new staff or resident cases.[50] Using this definition of an outbreak, we analyzed CDC's COVID-19 nursing home data for descriptive statistics, including the number and duration of nursing home outbreaks each nursing home experienced.

From June 14, 2020, through January 2, 2022, 15,281 nursing homes reported data to CDC and we found that those homes had a total of 102,992 outbreaks. Nursing homes had an average of 7.6 outbreaks and a median of eight outbreaks (2,435 nursing homes) over the review period, ranging from zero (25 nursing homes) to 16 (one nursing home) outbreaks. Forty-two percent of the outbreaks (43,753 of 102,992 outbreaks) lasted 1 week, with outbreak duration averaging 4 weeks (6,316 outbreaks) and ranging to 53 weeks (one outbreak).

Other Data Sources

We used additional data sources to create measures of independent variables for the regression analysis. In order to understand our universe

---

in this analysis are part of a live data set, meaning that facilities can correct the data at any time.

[50] See Centers for Disease Control and Prevention, *Interim Infection Prevention and Control Recommendations to Prevent SARS-CoV-2 Spread in Nursing Homes*, accessed September 7, 2022, https://www.cdc.gov/coronavirus/2019-ncov/hcp/long-term-care.html.

of nursing homes, we examined the descriptive information for each variable.

Nursing Home Characteristics

CMS's publicly available nursing home provider information file contains information on a number of characteristics, such as number of beds and non-profit or for-profit status, of nursing homes certified to participate in Medicare or Medicaid.[51] This file contained information on 15,622 nursing homes during our period of review. To determine whether a nursing home was located in a metropolitan or micropolitan core based statistical area, or neither, we merged the provider information file with Health Resources and Services Administration's publicly available county-level Area Health Resources Files.[52]

Using the merged file, we examined the breakdown of all Medicare- and Medicaid-certified nursing homes by facility characteristic for all categorical variables. (See Table 3). In addition, for two continuous variables, we calculated the average across all nursing homes, finding that nursing homes had an average of 106 beds and an average of 78 residents during our period of review.

Table 3. Nursing home facility characteristics, categorical variables, June 14, 2020, through January 2, 2022

Nursing home facility characteristics	Number of nursing homes (n = 15,622)	Percentage of nursing homes
Ownership type		
For-profit	10,651	68.2
Nonprofit	3,384	21.7
Government-owned	834	5.3
Mixed ownershipa	753	4.8

---

[51] The CMS publicly available nursing home provider information files were accessed on July 22, 2022, from https://data.cms.gov/provider-data/dataset/4pq5-n9py.

[52] The Health Resources and Services Administration publicly available 2020 and 2021 Area Health Resources Files (county-level data) were accessed on July 22, 2022, from https://data .hrsa.gov/data/download.

The Health Resources and Services Administration defines core based statistical areas as the following: (a) Metropolitan—at least one urbanized area of 50,000 or more population plus adjacent territory that has a high degree of social and economic integration with the core as measured by commuting ties; and (b) Micropolitan—at least one urban cluster of at least 10,000 but less than 50,000 population, plus adjacent territory that has a high degree of social and economic integration with the core as measured by commuting ties. We categorized all counties that did not meet the prior two criteria as rural.

Table 3. (Continued)

Nursing home facility characteristics	Number of nursing homes (n = 15,622)	Percentage of nursing homes
Certification type		
Medicare-only	667	4.3
Medicaid-only	348	2.2
Medicare and Medicaid	14,606	93.5
Facility type		
Hospital-based	699	4.5
Freestanding	14,923	95.6
*Location type*b		
Metropolitan	11,297	72.3
Micropolitan	2,144	13.7
Rural	2,173	13.9
Transitioning area	5	0
Change of ownership in last 12 months		
Home had a change of ownership	1,128	7.2
Home did not have a change of ownership	14,494	92.8
Average number of Medicare- and Medicaid-certified beds		
Less than 50 beds	1,946	12.5
50 to 99 beds	5,948	38.1
100 to 199 beds	6,834	43.8
200 or more beds	894	5.7
*Special Focus Facility status*c		
Special Focus Facility	68	0.4
Special Focus Facility candidate	975	6.2
Both Special Focus Facility home and candidate	101	0.6
Not a Special Focus Facility or candidate	14,478	92.7
*Continuing care residential community*d		
Continuing care residential community	1,872	12.0
Not a continuing care residential community	13,750	88.0
*Resident and family councils*e		
Resident council only	11,601	74.3
Family council only	28	0.2
Both resident and family councils	3,481	22.3
Separate resident council and family council	18	0.1
No resident or family councils	494	3.2
*Overall Five-Star rating*f		
Average rating of four or five stars	5,420	34.7
Average rating of three stars	3,308	21.2
Average rating of one or two stars	6,894	44.1
*Health inspections Five-Star rating*f		
Average rating of four or five stars	3,739	23.9
Average rating of three stars	3,645	23.3
Average rating of one or two stars	8,238	52.7
*Staffing Five-Star rating*f		
Average rating of four or five stars	3,571	22.9

Nursing home facility characteristics	Number of nursing homes (n = 15,622)	Percentage of nursing homes
Average rating of three stars	4,326	27.7
Average rating of one or two stars	7,725	49.5
*Quality measure Five-Star rating*f		
Average rating of four or five stars	7,371	47.2
Average rating of three stars	4,096	26.2
Average rating of one or two stars	4,155	26.6

Source: GAO analysis of Centers for Medicare & Medicaid Services data and the Health Resources and Services Administrations' Area Health Resources Files. | GAO-23-104291.

Notes: Percentages do not always add to 100 due to missing data and rounding. The percentage of nursing homes with missing data, if any, was less than 1 percent for each category.

[a] "Mixed ownership" refers to nursing homes that changed their ownership type at any point over the period of review.

[b] The Health Resources and Services Administration defines core based statistical areas as the following: (a) Metropolitan—at least one urbanized area of 50,000 or more population plus adjacent territory that has a high degree of social and economic integration with the core as measured by commuting ties; and (b) Micropolitan—at least one urban cluster of at least 10,000 but less than 50,000 population, plus adjacent territory that has a high degree of social and economic integration with the core as measured by commuting ties. We categorized all counties that did not meet the prior two criteria as rural. In addition, we considered a "transitioning area" to be a county where the statistical area designation changed at some point during the period of review.

[c] Nursing homes with chronic noncompliance with federal standards can be selected for the Special Focus Facility program, which requires state survey agencies to conduct more frequent oversight and the nursing homes to improve performance or risk termination from the Medicare and Medicaid programs.

[d] Continuing care resident communities offer multiple housing options and levels of care. A nursing home is typically the most service-intensive housing option. Residents may move from one level to another based on their particular needs, while typically still remaining in the community.

[e] Resident and family councils are usually organized and managed by nursing home residents or the residents' families to address concerns and improve the quality of care and life for the resident.

[f] The Five-Star Quality Rating System assigns each nursing home participating in the Medicare or Medicaid programs an overall "star" rating, ranging from one to five. Nursing homes with five stars are considered to have much above average quality, while nursing homes receiving one star are considered to have much below average quality. Calculation of the overall star rating is based on separate ratings that nursing homes receive for each of three components: health inspections, staffing, and quality measures. We calculated the average overall and component ratings for each nursing home during our period of review.

Nursing Home History of Infection Prevention and Control Deficiencies

CMS maintains data on nursing home surveys and deficiencies, including the dates of surveys and the number and type of deficiencies cited.[53] To determine

[53] In general, CMS requires that state survey agencies conduct standard surveys, or evaluations, approximately once each year of the state's nursing homes and investigate both complaints

the number of infection prevention and control deficiencies each nursing home received and the average number of these deficiencies cited per nursing home, we merged three different CMS datasets—the Certification and Survey Provider Enhanced Reports system data, the publicly available nursing home inspection dates file, and the publicly available nursing home health citations file.[54] (See Table 4). These files contained information on 13,614 nursing homes with deficiencies in 2017 and 12,343 nursing homes with deficiencies in 2021.

Table 4. Infection prevention and control deficiencies cited in nursing homes, by year, 2017 through 2021

Year	Number of surveyed nursing homes	Total number of infection prevention and control deficiencies	Average infection prevention and control deficiencies per surveyed nursing home
2017	14,184	6,527	0.5
2018	14,594	6,874	0.5
2019	14,776	6,913	0.5
2020	15,406	9,775	0.6
2021	14,128	6,738	0.5

Source: GAO analysis of Centers for Medicare & Medicaid Services data. | GAO-23-104291

Nursing Home Staffing

CMS's payroll-based journal collects employee-level payroll information for various types of nursing home staff, including registered nurses, licensed

from the public and facility-reported incidents regarding resident care or safety. Beginning in March 2020, CMS required state survey agencies to conduct focused infection control surveys, a new type of survey in response to the pandemic with a narrower scope than a standard survey. State survey agencies are required to perform focused infection control surveys for 20 percent of nursing homes in their state annually, prioritizing those facilities that report new COVID-19 cases and low vaccination rates. If a surveyor from a state survey agency determines that a nursing home violated a federal standard during a survey or investigation, a nursing home receives a deficiency code specific to that standard, known as a deficiency.

[54] For this analysis, we analyzed the deficiency code F-880 for nursing homes that were cited for not meeting federal standards for establishing and maintaining an infection prevention and control program. This code went into effect as part of CMS's restructuring of its deficiency codes on November 28, 2017, replacing a prior deficiency code that had been in effect for several years. For infection prevention and control deficiencies cited in 2017 prior to this restructuring, we used the prior code.
The CMS publicly available nursing home survey dates files were accessed on March 28, 2022, from https://data.cms.gov/provider-data/dataset/svdt-c123. The publicly available nursing home health citations files were accessed on April 12, 2022, from https://data.cms.gov/provider-data/dataset/r5ix-sfxw.

practical nurses, and nurse aides, from all Medicare- or Medicaid-certified nursing homes. This dataset included information from 15,419 nursing homes during our period of review.[55] Using the payroll- based journal data, we determined the daily staffing levels during our period of review for the 32 types of staff CMS requires nursing homes to report.[56] (See Table 5).

Table 5. Nursing home average daily staffing levels, June 14, 2020, through January 2, 2022

Type of staff	Minimum hours worked per day	Average hours worked per day	Maximum hours worked per day
Administrator	7.6	7.7	7.8
Medical director	2.6	2.9	3.3
Other physician	4.4	4.9	5.1
Physician assistant	5.2	5.9	6.3
Registered nurse director of nursing	7.8	7.9	8.0
Registered nurse with administrative duties	7.7	7.7	7.8
Registered nurse	8.3	8.4	8.5
Licensed practical nurse with administrative duties	7.9	8.0	8.1
Licensed practical nurse	8.5	8.6	8.7
Certified nurse aide	7.8	7.9	8.0
Nurse aide in training	7.3	7.6	7.8
Medication aide/technician	8.3	8.5	8.6
Nurse practitioner	5.7	6.0	6.1
Clinical nurse specialist	7.1	7.5	7.8
Pharmacist	3.4	3.8	4.2
Dietitian	6.7	6.8	7.0
Paid feeding assistant	6.9	7.1	7.3

[55] According to CMS officials, 878 nursing homes had data issues outside of their control from December 11, 2021, through December 31, 2021, possibly resulting in missing payroll data for that time period. CMS provided us with a list of the affected nursing homes, and 874 were in our database. We checked to see if those homes had staffing levels consistent with projections based on prior month and prior year data and we excluded any outbreaks that had incomplete data.

[56] Nursing homes must submit accurate information on direct-care staffing to CMS's payroll-based journal each quarter. This information must be based on payroll and other verifiable and auditable data. CMS allows nursing homes to submit staffing information for 40 different types of staff, including both nurse staff and non-nurse staff. However, the agency only requires reporting for the 32 types of direct-care staff. According to CMS, the remaining eight types of staff (dentist, podiatrist, vocational service worker, clinical laboratory service worker, diagnostic x-ray service worker, blood service worker, housekeeping service worker, other service worker) are voluntary for nursing homes to report because they either do not meet the definition of direct-care or are not paid by nursing homes, so CMS could not audit their data. Due to concerns with the reliability of the data for these eight types of staff, we did not include them in our analysis.

Table 5. (Continued)

Type of staff	Minimum hours worked per day	Average hours worked per day	Maximum hours worked per day
Occupational therapist	6.0	6.2	6.3
Occupational therapy assistant	6.2	6.4	6.5
Occupational therapy aide	6.7	6.9	7.1
Physical therapist	5.9	6.2	6.4
Physical therapy assistant	6.2	6.4	6.5
Physical therapy aide	6.6	6.7	6.8
Respiratory therapist	8.1	8.4	8.5
Respiratory therapy technician	8.1	8.5	8.8
Speech/language pathologist	5.1	5.5	5.7
Therapeutic recreation specialist	7.2	7.4	7.5
Qualified activities professional	7.4	7.6	7.7
Other activities staff	7.0	7.1	7.2
Qualified social worker	7.6	7.7	7.8
Other social worker	7.5	7.6	7.7
Mental health service worker	7.0	7.2	7.4

Source: GAO analysis of Centers for Medicare & Medicaid Services data. | GAO-23-104291.

Note: The 32 staff types listed in the table are those CMS requires nursing homes to report to its payroll-based journal.

Reported Nursing Home Staff Shortages during the COVID-19 Pandemic

Using CDC's COVID-19 nursing home data, discussed above, we determined the average number of weeks during our period of review that nursing homes reported facing staff shortages (See Table 6). The dataset included information reported from 15,466 nursing homes during our period of review.

Table 6. Reported nursing home staff shortages during the COVID-19 pandemic, June 14, 2020, through January 2, 2022

Types of reported staffing shortages	Average number of weeks nursing homes reported shortage
Shortage of nursing staff	14.1
Shortage of clinical staff	1.8
Shortage of aides	15.8
Shortage of other staff	8.0

Source: GAO analysis of Centers for Disease Control and Prevention data. | GAO-23-104291.

Resident Demographics

CMS's Minimum Data Set collects information on each resident's strengths and needs, as well as resident demographic information, through regular comprehensive assessments conducted by all nursing homes certified to participate in Medicare or Medicaid.[57] The dataset included information for 15,416 nursing homes during our period of review. Using admission, quarterly, and annual assessments in the Minimum Data Set, we determined the average demographic makeup of all Medicare- and Medicaid-certified nursing homes during our period of review. (See Table 7). We also determined each nursing home's case-mix—that is, a numeric representation of the acuity of residents within a nursing home—using CMS's methodology.[58] We found that the total average case-mix score in nursing homes was 43.8, ranging from 0.5 to 568.9.

Table 7. Nursing home resident demographics, June 14, 2020, through January 2, 2022

Nursing home resident demographics	Percentage of residents within a nursing home
Resident age	
Less than 50	3.1
50 to less than 65	13.7
65 to less than 75	22.4
75 to less than 85	30.0
Greater than 85	30.8
Resident gender	
Male	
Female	
Resident race and ethnicity	
White	75.1
Black or African American	12.7
Hispanic or Latino	5.1
Asian	1.8

[57] The CMS Minimum Data Set is reported by nursing homes, which are required to complete resident assessments at regular intervals as part of federal requirements to participate in the Medicare and Medicaid programs. Nursing homes are required to conduct resident assessments at entry, quarterly, at discharge, and if there are any significant changes or corrections. During standard surveys, surveyors can evaluate whether a nursing home's assessments meet federal standards for accuracy.

[58] We used CMS's methodology to calculate the numeric case-mix index value associated with the resource utilization group obtained from non-therapy index maximizing classification.

Table 7. (Continued)

Native Hawaiian or Other Pacific Islander	0.2
American Indian or Alaska Native	0.4
Mixed ethnicity	0.4
Unknown	4.7

Source: GAO analysis of Centers for Medicare & Medicaid Services data. | GAO-23-104291.
Note: Percentages do not always add to 100 due to rounding.

Community Conditions during the COVID-19 Pandemic

CDC county-level COVID-19 community transmission data contain the daily levels of community transmission by county, known as community spread. The dataset included information on 3,222 counties. Using this data, we analyzed the number of weeks during our period of review that the level of COVID-19 community spread in each county was categorized by CDC as high, substantial, moderate, or low[59] (See Table 8).

Table 8. Number of weeks counties were designated by CDC as having high, substantial, moderate, or low levels of community transmission of COVID-19, June 14, 2020, through January 2, 2022

CDC levels of community spread	Minimum number of weeks	Average number of weeks	Maximum number of weeks
High	0	50.0	80.4
Substantial	0	11.9	37.0
Moderate	0	13.4	41.7
Low	0	6.7	82.0

Source: GAO analysis of Centers for Disease Control and Prevention (CDC) data. | GAO-23-104291.
Note: CDC calculated the level of community transmission using two indicators: (1) the total new cases per 100,000 persons within the last 7 days and (2) the percentage of positive diagnostic and screening nucleic acid amplification tests during the last 7 days. If the two indicators suggest

[59] CDC calculated the level of community transmission using two indicators: (1) the total new cases per 100,000 persons within the last 7 days and (2) the percentage of positive diagnostic and screening nucleic acid amplification tests during the last 7 days. If the two indicators suggest different transmission levels, the higher level is selected. Possible transmission categories are high (counties with 100 or more cumulative cases per 100,000 population or a cumulative test positivity result of 10.0 percent or higher in the past 7 days), substantial (counties with 50-99 cumulative cases per 100,000 population or a cumulative test positivity result between 8.0-9.9 percent in the past 7 days), moderate (counties with 10-49 cumulative cases per 100,000 population or a cumulative test positivity result between 5.0-7.9 percent in the past 7 days), or low (counties with fewer than 10 cumulative cases per 100,000 population in the past 7 days and a cumulative percent test positivity result below 5 percent in the past 7 days).

different transmission levels, the higher level is selected. Possible transmission categories are high (counties with 100 or more cumulative cases per 100,000 population or a cumulative test positivity result of 10.0 percent or higher in the past 7 days), substantial (counties with 50-99 cumulative cases per 100,000 population or a cumulative test positivity result between 8.0-9.9 percent in the past 7 days), moderate (counties with 10-49 cumulative cases per 100,000 population or a cumulative test positivity result between 5.0-7.9 percent in the past 7 days), or low (counties with fewer than 10 cumulative cases per 100,000 population in the past 7 days and a cumulative percent test positivity result below 5 percent in the past 7 days).

Analyzing the Data

We merged the CDC COVID-19 nursing home data with the data sets described in the sections above, creating a single analytic data file for our study period of June 14, 2020, through January 2, 2022.

Exclusions

We merged the data using weekly COVID-19 outbreaks as our unit of analysis. First, we excluded 117 nursing homes that had 50 weeks or more of CDC COVID-19 nursing home data that was missing or did not pass quality control. Second, we excluded 24 nursing homes that did not have data in CMS's publicly available data files. This resulted in a total of 15,322 nursing homes with 100,780 outbreaks. Third, we excluded 4,632 outbreaks due to missing data in CMS's Minimum Data Set, CMS's payroll-based journal, or both. All other data files were complete and did not result in any exclusions. After these exclusions, our analytic file included 15,091 nursing homes that had a total of 96,148 COVID-19 outbreaks.

Factors Not Included in Analysis

We could not control for all factors that may be associated with COVID-19 outbreak duration in nursing homes, often due to inconsistent data, incomplete data, or a lack of data entirely. Some examples include the following.

- *Equipment shortages.* We have reported on the lack of COVID-19 tests and personal protective equipment in nursing homes, particularly during the first year of the pandemic.[60] However, while CDC collected information from nursing homes on these types of shortages in its COVID-19 nursing home data, these variables were inconsistent across our period of review. For example, after the week

[60] See GAO-20-701, 129; GAO-21-191, 67; and GAO-21-265, 63.

ending on March 7, 2021, CDC removed questions related to whether nursing homes had any supply or a one week supply of personal protective equipment and added in similar, but slightly different questions, making it difficult to track consistently over time.

- *Vaccination rates.* The development and subsequent availability of COVID-19 vaccines for nursing home residents and staff at the end of 2020 was an important milestone in the pandemic, which corresponded with dramatic decreases in nursing home cases and deaths through the first part of 2021. However, nationwide data on the rate of vaccinations within each nursing home is incomplete—reporting was not required until May 2021—so we could not include these data as a variable in our regression. Instead, we ran two separate models to account for the time period before the introduction of vaccines and the time period after the introduction of vaccines. This is explained further in the following section.
- *State and local policies.* States and localities varied throughout the pandemic on what, if any, COVID-19 policies, such as masking requirements or the closure of non-essential businesses, they had in place. However, even when policies were in place, we could not quantify how well communities surrounding a nursing home enforced or complied with the policies. Therefore, rather than assess the reliability of data on state and local COVID-19 policies, we assumed that analyzing the effect of transmission of COVID-19 in the county where each nursing home is located would reflect both the local policies and the community's compliance with the policies.
- *Adherence to infection prevention and control practices.* We have previously reported on the importance of infection prevention and control practices and CDC continues to emphasize the importance of rigorous infection prevention and control to prevent the spread of COVID-19 in nursing homes.[61] Because CMS collects data on nursing home deficiencies, we were able to control for a nursing home's history of infection prevention and control deficiencies; however, we could not account for the day-to-day adherence by nursing home staff and residents to infection prevention and control practices.

---

[61] See GAO-22-105133.

Multivariate Regression Model

We conducted a series of multivariate Cox proportional hazard regression models. The purpose of the model is to evaluate simultaneously the effect of several factors on outbreak duration. A hazard regression model allows us to examine how specified factors may be associated with the rate of a particular event happening (e.g., outbreak ending) at a particular point in time and allows time-varying covariates to capture the effects of changes in independent variables over time.[62] The rate is commonly referred to as the hazard rate. Predictor variables (or independent factors) are usually termed covariates in the survival-analysis literature. The Cox model is expressed by the hazard function denoted by $\lambda(t)$. Briefly, the hazard function can be interpreted as the probability of the outbreak ending at time t. It can be estimated as follow:

$$\lambda_k(t; Z_{ki}) = \lambda_{k0} \exp\{\beta'_k Z_{ki}(t)\}$$

where

- k is the event, which in our case is the outbreak ($k = 1, \ldots, K$).
- i is the subject, which in our case is the nursing home ($i = 1, \ldots, n$).
- Z represents the set of covariates. Z_{ki} represents the specific covariate associated with ki.
- $\lambda_{k0}(t)$ is the baseline hazard function (hazard rate at time t).
- $\exp\{\beta'_k Z_{ki}(t)\}$ is the expected hazard ratio of covariates at time (t).

The value of $\exp(\beta)$ is the hazard ratio. A value of β greater than zero, or equivalently a hazard ratio greater than one, indicates that as the value of the covariate increases, the hazard increases and thus the duration of the outbreak decreases.

Multivariate regression modeling is a statistical method that examines multiple variables simultaneously to estimate whether each of these variables are more likely or less likely to be associated with a certain outcome, controlling for the other variables. A multivariate regression analyzes the statistical influence of each individual factor with the outcome. This type of modeling allowed us to test the association between nursing home factors,

[62] We did not use a hierarchical model on top of an already complex model. A hierarchical model would help to account for potential correlation between outbreak durations within the same nursing home. When we checked for this potential correlation in an hierarchical model with no other factors included, we found there was no significant correlation between outbreak durations within the same nursing home.

such as nursing home size or nursing home ownership, and the probability (hazard rate) of the COVID-19 outbreak ending, while holding other nursing home information constant (such as staffing levels and resident demographics as independent variables).

A Cox proportional hazard model provides an estimated hazard ratio for each independent variable, where a value greater than one indicates a higher likelihood of the COVID-19 outbreak ending (the dependent, or outcome, variable) and an estimated hazard ratio less than one indicates lower probability of the outbreak ending, controlling for all the other independent variables. For example, an overall staffing level with an estimated hazard ratio of 2.0 would indicate a higher probability of an outbreak ending. In contrast, an overall staffing level with an estimated staffing ratio of 0.5 would indicate a higher probability that the outbreak continues.

The statistical significance of the results for each variable is determined by a p-value of less than 0.05. As a result, in our report, we state that hazard ratios that are statistically significant and greater than 1.00 or lower than 1.00 indicate that nursing homes with that characteristic (e.g., rural location) are more likely or less likely, respectively, to have their COVID-19 outbreak end at that point in time, relative to their corresponding reference category. In cases where the p-value was greater than 0.05, we report that we could not identify any statistically significant differences, which means that we could not conclude that there was an association between that attribute and the likelihood of the outbreak ending.

Table 9. Multivariate regression results from Cox proportional hazard model, COVID-19 outbreak duration by vaccination time period, June 14, 2020, through January 2, 2022

	Hazard ratio (parameter estimate)	
Independent factors	Pre-vaccine time period (June 14, 2020, through January 2, 2021)	Post-vaccine time period (January 3, 2021, through January 2, 2022)
Categorical variables		
Reference category: High community spread		
Low community spread	2.784** (1.024)	1.999** (0.692)
Moderate community spread	2.382** (0.868)	1.920** (0.652)
Substantial community spread	2.014** (0.700)	1.703** (0.533)
Reference category: Metropolitan		
Rural	1.023 (0.023)	1.042* (0.041)
Micropolitan	0.978 (-0.022)	0.990 (-0.010)
Reference category: Large (100 – 199 beds) or very large (200 or more beds)		

Independent factors	Pre-vaccine time period (June 14, 2020, through January 2, 2021)	Post-vaccine time period (January 3, 2021, through January 2, 2022)
Medium (50 to <100 beds)	1.177** (0.163)	1.167** (0.155)
Small (<50 beds)	1.444** (0.367)	1.414** (0.346)
Reference category: For-profit		
Non-profit	0.882** (-0.125)	0.884** (-0.124)
Government-owned	0.903** (-0.102)	0.799** (-0.225)
Reference category: No reported staff shortages		
Reported staff shortages	0.843** (-0.170)	0.944** (-0.058)
Reference category: Lower overall star rating (one- to three-stars)		
Higher overall star rating (four- and five-stars)	0.933** (-0.070)	0.956** (-0.045)
Reference category: Lower health inspection star rating (one- to three-stars)		
Higher health inspection star rating (four- and five- stars)	1.004 (0.004)	1.006 (0.006)
Continuous variables		
Number of prior outbreaks	0.959** (-0.042)	1.074** (0.072)
Percentage of new employeesa	0.987** (-0.013)	1.003** (0.003)
Average hours per employee per week	0.996 (-0.004)	1.000 (0.000)
Number of employees per resident	0.984 (-0.016)	0.969** (-0.031)
Nursing home case-mix	0.995** (-0.005)	0.995** (-0.005)
Percentage of occupied beds	1.001 (0.001)	0.999** (-0.001)
Number of infection prevention and control deficiencies cited in the last year	0.955** (-0.046)	1.006 (0.006)
Percentage of residents over 75	1.001 (0.001)	1.001 (0.001)
Percentage of residents less than 65	1.005* (0.005)	1.006** (0.006)
Percentage of female residents	1.001 (0.001)	1.002** (0.002)
Percentage of minority residents	1.001** (0.001)	1.001* (0.001)

Legend:

"*" indicates that this variable is statistically significant at p-value <0.05.

"**" indicates that this variable is statistically significant at p-value <0.001.

Source: GAO analysis of Centers for Disease Control and Prevention, Centers for Medicare & Medicaid Services (CMS), and Health Resources and Services Administration data. | GAO-23-104291.

Notes: Multivariate Cox Proportional Hazard models are used to test the extent of association with outcome and statistical significance of all independent factors.

The hazard ratio is the probability of an outbreak ending for the given factor relative to its reference category. In our report, we state that hazard ratios that are statistically significant and greater than 1.00 or lower than 1.00 indicate that nursing homes with that characteristic are more likely or less likely, respectively, to have their COVID-19 outbreak end at that point in time.

The parameter estimate is the measure of the direction and size of the effect that a single unit change in the independent variable has on the dependent variable. The parameter estimate is based on weekly data (parameter estimate of 1.00 equals 1 week); therefore, a parameter estimate of approximately +/- 0.143 is equivalent to one day.

[a]New employees were defined as any employee at a specific nursing home without a record in CMS's payroll-based journal in the prior 6 weeks.

We developed multivariate Cox proportional hazard models to test the extent of association with outcome and statistical significance of all independent factors presented in Table 9.[63] We ran two models—one for the period of time prior to the introduction of COVID-19 vaccines (June 14, 2020, through January 2, 2021) and one for the period of time after introduction of COVID-19 vaccines in nursing homes (January 3, 2021, through January 2, 2022).[64] Hazard ratios from the multivariate model represent simultaneous relationships of all independent factors specified in the model with the outcome. Therefore, there is a reference category for each categorical factor specified in the multivariate model. As an example, for nursing home size, small and medium nursing homes are compared against large and very large nursing homes as the reference category in the model. Based on the results in Table 9, in the pre-vaccine time period, small nursing homes had a statistically significant hazard ratio of 1.444, indicating that small homes were distinct from large and very large homes and that the small homes had shorter outbreaks than larger homes. Further, the parameter estimate of 0.367 indicates that an outbreak was likely to end approximately 2.5 days earlier in small homes than in large and very large homes.

Data and Model Limitations

Although the data quality is sufficiently reliable for the purposes of our objective, there are some limitations to note. The CDC COVID-19 nursing home data, which forms the backbone of the COVID-19 outbreak variable and other variables, is self-reported weekly by nursing homes. The number of COVID-19 cases is based on the testing technology and infrastructure available to homes at the time the data were reported; the availability and accuracy of the tests may have changed over time, but there is no reason to believe that any bias in testing occurred between homes at the time. In addition, according to CDC officials, the agency's definition of a COVID-19 outbreak is an epidemiologic one and has been used during the pandemic to trigger the implementation of additional infection prevention and control practices, such as screening testing for residents and staff to determine if unrecognized cases were in the nursing home. Therefore, an individual outbreak in our analysis does not necessarily imply that all of the COVID-19

[63] The model results presented are right-censored.

[64] We initially ran a single model with a dummy variable for the time period that COVID-19 vaccinations were available but found that this dummy variable was overly dominate. Therefore, by running two separate models we were able to tease out the effects of other independent variables.

cases reported during that outbreak were related to a single introduction of COVID-19 into the facility.

CDC officials also noted that the inclusion of staff COVID-19 cases in our analysis of outbreaks may inflate the total number and duration of outbreaks because routine screening testing of asymptomatic nursing home staff could have identified infected staff who may have never entered the facility. This situation would reflect COVID-19 transmission in the community rather than transmission in the nursing home.

Other variables in the COVID-19 nursing home data weekly reports, such as the availability of staffing and personal protective equipment, are also self-reported. While noting the staffing shortages are self-reported, we also included CMS payroll-based journal data that provide an objective measure of staffing. In the case of personal protective equipment and infection containment supplies (such as hand sanitizer), CDC altered the questions at different periods during the pandemic. This resulted in data that could not be tracked over time and thus we did not include variables on personal protective equipment shortages in the final models. The vaccination of staff and residents posed a slightly different problem, in that CMS did not require nursing homes to report data to CDC on the number and percent of staff and residents vaccinated until about 5 months into the vaccination program. To account for the possible role that the presence of the vaccine played in COVID-19 outbreaks, we first created a dummy variable to acknowledge the availability of the vaccine. When this proved to be an overwhelmingly significant variable, we split the model into two time periods, as described above.

Other datasets also had limitations. In its payroll-based journal CMS allows nursing homes to submit staffing information for 40 different types of staff, including both nurse and non-nurse staff. While CMS has instituted checks and audits to ensure that nurse staffing data reported in the payroll-based journal are accurate, CMS does not have a process to ensure the accuracy and completeness of staffing information for non-nurse staff.[65] Based on interviews with CMS officials, we determined that, despite this limitation, we could still use most of the non-nurse payroll- based journal data

[65] The Department of Health and Human Services' Office of Inspector General has recommended that CMS take steps to ensure the accuracy of payroll-based journal data for non-nurse staff that it chooses to include on its Care Compare website. For example, CMS may consider adding physical therapists—the only type of non-nurse staff with data currently found on Care Compare—to its audits of payroll-based journal data. See Department of Health and Human Services Office of Inspector General, *CMS Use of Data on Nursing Home Staffing: Progress and Opportunities To Do More*, OEI-04-18-00451 (Washington, D.C.: March 2021).

for the purposes of our analysis. However, CMS only requires reporting for 32 of the 40 types of staff. Data for the remaining eight types of non-nurse staff—which include housekeepers and others who may not care for residents in a therapeutic manner but still may come into close contact with residents—are neither required to be reported nor audited for accuracy.[66] As a result, we decided to exclude these eight types of staff from our analysis. Therefore, we do not know if these types of staff were associated with the duration of outbreaks.

When using staffing variables created based on data in the payroll-based journal, we were generally not able to separate out the influence of certain staff roles (e.g., registered nurses and nurse aides) to our satisfaction. While many of the homes we interviewed pointed to staffing as an issue, the actual employment data, despite several different iterations using different breakouts of staffing roles, did not indicate a significant role by particular kinds of staff.

CDC data on community spread is based on test results. While there is no imputation that accounts for cases that exist but for which no test was done or tests were done at home and not reported, we used CDC's categorization of community spread, which is based, in part, on the percentage of positive diagnostic and screening nucleic acid amplification tests, which are required to be reported. CDC data is assumed to be reliable for our purposes because we can assume that there was no systematic bias with respect to the duration of outbreaks in nursing homes.

In general, CMS data on nursing home surveys and investigations and their resulting deficiencies is considered reliable. We should note that for a number of months during the first year of the pandemic, regular standard surveys of nursing homes and low priority investigations were temporarily suspended, replaced by focused infection control surveys, which evaluated compliance with CMS infection prevention and control policies. Based on this and findings in prior reports we focused on a home's history of infection prevention and control deficiencies rather than on their overall number and severity of deficiencies.

The CMS Minimum Data Set was used to determine the case-mix of the residents in a home as well as the demographics of each home's population. Many variables within the Minimum Data Set are self-reported by the resident,

---

[66] According to CMS, these eight types of staff (dentist, podiatrist, vocational service worker, clinical laboratory service worker, diagnostic x-ray service worker, blood service worker, housekeeping service worker, other service worker) are voluntary for nursing homes to report because they either do not meet the definition of direct-care or are not paid by nursing homes, so their data would not be able to be audited by CMS.

the family, or a staff member on behalf of a resident, and we acknowledge this can raise some questions of data reliability, some of which have been reported in the literature.[67] We determined that the demographic data are sufficiently reliable. Further, we determined that case-mix data are sufficiently reliable given that any bias in case-mix is likely to exist in all nursing homes, so comparison of homes is not particularly problematic.

Appendix III: Nursing Home Officials' Descriptions of COVID-19 Outbreaks, including Challenges and Successes

Table 10. Nursing home officials' descriptions of COVID-19 outbreaks, including challenges and successes

Nursing home	Description of COVID-19 outbreaks, including challenges and successes
Nursing home A *Non-profit* *Large* *(100-199 beds)*	This nursing home kept COVID-19 out of the facility until July 2020, which was likely due to the proactive steps it took to restrict residents to their rooms and adopt face mask requirements. Their first case was a staff member, and it was caught early. The required biweekly COVID-19 testing caught additional staff cases throughout the pandemic. The challenges posed by the reduction in staff due to quarantine or symptoms was "manageable although not optimal." However, the home reached a staffing "crisis" as the pandemic continued, noting that they were down 25 full-time employees. The nursing home's first resident outbreak was in October 2020 and started with five residents and then spread to an additional 16 residents. The nursing home officials believed that COVID-19 entered the home from a dialysis patient. The COVID-positive residents were able to be isolated in one ward of the nursing home and staff who already had tested positive and had returned from their quarantine were willing to work in the COVID-19 unit. A year later, in October 2021, the home had a second "major" resident outbreak.
Nursing home B *For-profit* *Large* *(100-199 beds)*	This nursing home experienced its largest outbreak in December 2021 with the Omicron surge. During this time, 20 percent of its residents and staff tested positive. Officials attributed this outbreak in part to the re-opening of visitation that occurred in November 2021. Prior to the outbreak, the home had only seen a few cases at a time, and its COVID-19-positive residents had avoided severe illness. A lot of the home's prior success in keeping COVID-19 out of the facility was due to community decisions that resulted in low levels of COVID-19. Located

[67] Some studies have found that the Minimum Data Set data reported by nursing homes underreports anti-psychotic use and falls. For examples, see HHS Office of Inspector General, *CMS Could Improve the Data It Uses to Monitor Antipsychotic Drugs in Nursing Homes*, OEI-07-19-00490 (Washington, D.C.: May 3, 2021), and J. Mintz et al., "Validation of the Minimum Data Set Items on Falls and Injury in Two Long-Stay Facilities," *Journal of the American Geriatrics Society*, vol. 69, no. 4 (April 2021).

Table 10. (Continued)

Nursing home	Description of COVID-19 outbreaks, including challenges and successes
	in an isolated area, the county was able to close a road into the community during the worst of the pandemic in 2020 to keep travelers out. However, these community policies were discontinued by winter of 2021, and the nursing home could no longer restrict visitation. Officials also discussed staffing shortages and staff fatigue as challenges experienced during outbreaks. For example, at one point the home was down five working staff members as COVID-19-positive staff had to quarantine. In addition, the home had to staff a separate COVID-19 unit for just a few COVID-19-positive residents during a smaller outbreak, requiring more staff. It was also difficult to find staff willing to work the COVID-19 unit due to the risk of exposure.
Nursing home C *For-profit* *Very large* *(200+ beds)*	This nursing home kept COVID-19 out of the facility until May 2020, which the home attributed to having enough personal protective equipment, suspending new admissions, and adopting face mask requirements. But mitigation measures only worked for a while. The first of two resident outbreaks started with a few staff contracting COVID-19 from the community. Soon after, two residents tested positive, then two more, and so on. During the first outbreak, the virus spread slowly, but the second outbreak in late 2020 spread more rapidly—from two residents to 10 or 12 residents almost immediately. During the first outbreak, the boundaries of the COVID-19 unit never changed, but during the second outbreak the home had to keep expanding the boundaries. Throughout the outbreaks, the nursing home was able to maintain its staffing levels—even when staff were out sick with COVID-19. However, the psychosocial toll had significant negative effects on residents. The suspension not only of visitation but also dining facility activities resulted in declines in resident physical and mental health. The staff began to see residents with weight loss and an increased need for anti-depressant drugs. Many of the residents just "gave up."
Nursing home D *Non-profit* *Very large* *(200+ beds)*	This nursing home was hit "like a brick" in the fall of 2020. Earlier in 2020, a COVID-19 outbreak affected about a dozen residents, but cases in its outbreak in the fall of 2020 "wreaked havoc" on residents and staff, with 40 residents dying. The loss of so many residents took a heavy emotional toll on staff and fellow residents. Officials believed the virus entered the facility through staff as, at the time, the home's staff and the surrounding community had low vaccination rates. In addition to the emotional toll on residents and staff, the number of resident deaths plus staff attrition resulted in the nursing home losing about 50 percent of its capacity and closing a sister nursing home. The home learned a lot about the importance of communication during the second outbreak. For example, to facilitate communication within the home, task force teams met twice a week, and to facilitate communication to families, a hotline was created and a weekly newsletter was developed to provide relevant COVID-19 information. However, the psychosocial toll during that time took the joy away from caregiving and left many staff with trauma.

Nursing home	Description of COVID-19 outbreaks, including challenges and successes
	Further, the fact that the home is located in a rural area with limited available staff, made maintaining staffing levels very difficult, with officials noting "scary" staffing shortages.
Nursing home E *For-profit* *Medium* *(50-99 beds)*	This nursing home kept COVID-19 out of the facility until July 2020 and used its outbreak-free time learning to adapt to infection control procedures that very few staff were doing correctly before the pandemic. The July 2020 outbreak lasted about 5 weeks and culminated with 32 of about 70 residents and 12 staff infected. Eight of those residents died. After that outbreak, the nursing home did not experience any additional large outbreaks, only a few isolated cases. Officials could not trace the origin of the outbreak, but believed that COVID-19 was brought into the facility by a staff member. Further exacerbating the outbreak was a limited supply of N95 masks, so many residents and some staff were using regular procedure masks instead, as well as physical space constraints. Officials said that to isolate COVID-19-positive residents, the home had to "shuffle" healthy residents from one room to another, which may have accidentally spread the virus. In addition, the nursing home's resident population and nurse staff decreased significantly. Specifically, the nursing home lost 23 residents and about half of its staff left. This resulted in closing a section of the home in December 2020 and having to rely on traveling nurses and aides for the home's staffing needs.
Nursing home F *For-profit* *Large* *(100-199 beds)*	Early in the pandemic, this nursing home had some staff members test positive, but COVID-19 was not transferred to the residents. The first resident did not test positive until November 2020. Officials believed that the virus was brought into the facility by staff. The home had another outbreak in January 2021 and was able to contain COVID to just one floor of their three-floor facility for a time, but eventually the virus spread. Staff were out sick with COVID-19 during these outbreaks. With limited staff and the building's physical space constraints, officials had to make difficult choices. For example, there were times where nursing home officials felt they had no choice but to move staff between COVID-19 and non-COVID-19 units. As the pandemic wore on, staff had a hard time adjusting to the re-opening of visitation in November 2021. Officials said that they believed their staff were exposed to trauma as a result of their early experiences with COVID-19.

Source: GAO interviews with officials from selected nursing homes in four states. | GAO-23-104291.

Chapter 4

COVID-19 in Nursing Homes: CMS Needs to Continue to Strengthen Oversight of Infection Prevention and Control*

United States Government Accountability Office

Abbreviations

CDC	Centers for Disease Control and Prevention
CMS	Centers for Medicare & Medicaid Services
HHS	Department of Health and Human Services
IPC	Infection Prevention and Control

Why GAO Did This Study

Implementing proper infection prevention and control practices can be critical for preventing the spread of infectious diseases. Infection prevention and control has been a long-standing concern in the nation's more than 15,000 nursing homes—one that the COVID-19 pandemic has brought into sharper focus. Some infection prevention and control practices in nursing homes, such as social isolation, may negatively affect resident mental and physical health.

The CARES Act directs GAO to monitor the federal pandemic response. GAO was also asked to review federal oversight of nursing homes in light of

* This is an edited, reformatted and augmented version of the United States Government Accountability Office Report to Congressional Addressees, Publication No. GAO-22-105133, dated September 2022.

In: COVID-19 in Nursing Homes
Editor: Fred C. Wallace
ISBN: 979-8-88697-673-1

the pandemic. Among other objectives, this report: (1) describes what data reveal about any changes in resident health before and during the pandemic and (2) examines infection prevention and control actions CMS and CDC have taken in nursing homes before and during the pandemic.

GAO (1) reviewed CMS and CDC documents, (2) analyzed CMS resident health data from 2018 through 2021, and (3) interviewed CMS, CDC, state survey agency, and nursing home officials in a non-generalizable sample of eight states selected for variation in factors such as geographic location.

What GAO Recommends

GAO is making three recommendations to CMS related to the role of the infection preventionist and clarifying infection prevention and control guidance. HHS agreed with our first recommendation, but neither agreed nor disagreed with our other two recommendations.

What GAO Found

The Centers for Medicare & Medicaid Services (CMS) is responsible for ensuring that nursing homes meet federal standards. CMS enters into agreements with state survey agencies to conduct surveys and investigations of the state's nursing homes. The Centers for Disease Control and Prevention (CDC) issues guidance, operates surveillance systems, and provides technical assistance to support infection prevention and control in nursing homes.

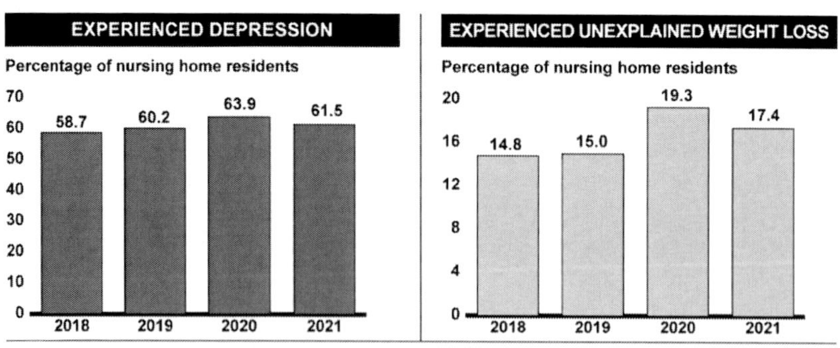

Source: GAO analysis of Centers for Medicare and Medicaid Services (CMS) data. | GAO-22-105133.

GAO analysis of CMS data reported by nursing homes shows that seven of the eight key indicators of nursing home resident mental and physical health worsened at least slightly the first year of the pandemic (2020), compared to the years prior to the pandemic. See the figure below for examples of two outcomes we reviewed.

CMS and CDC took actions on infection prevention and control prior to and during the COVID-19 pandemic. For example, prior to the pandemic, CMS required nursing homes to designate an infection preventionist on staff. This person is a trained employee responsible for the home's infection prevention and control program and was crucial to nursing homes during the pandemic. CMS also made changes in how nursing homes were surveyed during the pandemic. However, GAO found areas where CMS could take additional actions, including:

- Strengthening oversight of the infection preventionist role. GAO identified ways CMS could strengthen oversight of the infection preventionist role, such as by establishing minimum training standards. CMS could also collect infection preventionist staffing data and use it to determine whether the current infection preventionist staffing requirement is sufficient.
- Strengthening infection prevention and control guidance. GAO identified how CMS could strengthen this guidance by providing information to help surveyors assess the scope and severity of infection prevention and control deficiencies they identify. For example, CMS could add COVID-19-relevant examples for scope and severity classifications to its State Operations Manual—the key guidance state survey agencies use for conducting nursing home surveys.

Letter

September 14, 2022

Congressional Addressees

Infection prevention and control (IPC) has been a long-standing concern in the nation's more than 15,000 Medicare- and Medicaid-certified nursing homes—

one the COVID-19 pandemic has brought into sharper focus.[1] Prior to the COVID-19 pandemic, infections were a leading cause of death and hospitalization among nursing home residents, with estimates of up to 380,000 residents dying each year.[2] Since that time, COVID-19 has emerged as a new and highly contagious respiratory disease that has had devastating consequences for the nation's more than one million nursing home residents, including high rates of severe illness and death. COVID-19 has also substantially affected the broader nursing home industry, including nursing home staff. The initial unknown nature of the virus that causes COVID-19 and the scope of the pandemic also created unprecedented challenges for state and federal agencies that work to ensure the quality of care delivered in nursing homes and to protect public health.[3]

In our previous reporting, we found that, in the years prior to the pandemic, nursing homes had persistent and widespread challenges with IPC.[4] For example, we found that implementing proper IPC practices, such as isolating infected residents, can be critical for preventing the spread of infectious diseases, including COVID-19—thus protecting both resident and staff health and well-being. However, some IPC practices in nursing homes, such as social isolation, may negatively affect resident mental and physical health.[5]

The Department of Health and Human Services (HHS), primarily through the Centers for Medicare & Medicaid Services (CMS) and the Centers for Disease Control and Prevention (CDC), has led the response to the COVID-19 pandemic in nursing homes. CMS is the federal oversight agency responsible for ensuring that nursing homes meet federal quality standards to be eligible to participate in the Medicare and Medicaid programs. These

---

[1] According to the Centers for Disease Control and Prevention, IPC protects patients, residents, healthcare personnel, and visitors by preventing healthcare-associated infections and limiting the spread of pathogens through the implementation of evidence-based interventions.

[2] Department of Health and Human Services, The National Action Plan to Prevent Health Care-Associated Infections: Road Map to Elimination (Washington, D.C.: 2013).

[3] As GAO has previously reported, during the COVID-19 pandemic, nursing homes experienced high staff cases and deaths and challenges related to staffing, personal protective equipment, and testing. See, for example, GAO, *COVID-19: Federal Efforts Could Be Strengthened by Timely and Concerted Actions*, GAO-20-701 (Washington, D.C.: Sept. 21, 2020).

[4] GAO, *Infection Control Deficiencies Were Widespread and Persistent in Nursing Homes Prior to COVID-19 Pandemic*, GAO-20-576R (Washington, D.C.: May 20, 2020).

[5] National Academies of Sciences, Engineering, and Medicine, Social Isolation and Loneliness in Older Adults: Opportunities for the Health Care System (Washington, D.C.: The National Academies Press, 2020).

standards require, for example, that nursing homes establish and maintain an IPC program. To monitor compliance with these standards, CMS enters into agreements with state survey agencies in each state government and oversees the work the state survey agencies do. CDC issues guidance with recommendations for preventing and managing infectious diseases, operates infectious disease surveillance systems, and provides technical assistance through programs aimed at supporting and assessing IPC in nursing homes, and tracking IPC data.

The CARES Act includes a provision directing us to monitor the federal response to the COVID-19 pandemic.[6] Further, you also asked us to examine federal oversight of IPC protocols and the adequacy of emergency preparedness standards for emerging infectious diseases in nursing homes, as well as CMS's response to the pandemic. Since 2020, we have examined the response to COVID-19 in nursing homes in multiple studies. Some studies have been completed and released and others are ongoing. (See app. I for a list of completed related reports.)

In this report, we: (1) describe what data reveal about any changes in resident mental and physical health before and during the COVID -19 pandemic, (2) describe whether IPC challenges have persisted in nursing homes during the pandemic, and (3) examine the IPC actions that CMS and CDC have taken related to nursing homes before and during the pandemic.

To describe what data reveal about any changes in resident mental and physical health before and during the COVID-19 pandemic, we analyzed 2018 through 2021 CMS Minimum Data Set resident assessment data.[7] We compared selected health indicators across calendar years for all long-stay residents who had lived in the nursing home greater than 100 days.[8] We selected four mental and four physical health indicators to analyze based on

---

[6] Pub. L. No. 116-136, § 19010(b), 134 Stat. 281, 580 (2020). Throughout the pandemic, we regularly issued government-wide reports on the federal response to COVID-19. All government-wide reports are available on GAO's website at https://www.gao.gov/coronavirus.

[7] 72021 was the most recent calendar year available at the time of our analysis. The CMS Minimum Data Set is reported by nursing homes, which are required to complete resident assessments at regular intervals as part of federal requirements to participate in the Medicare and Medicaid programs. Nursing homes are required to conduct resident assessments at entry, quarterly, at discharge, and if there are any significant changes or corrections. During standard surveys, surveyors can evaluate whether a nursing home's assessments meet federal standards for accuracy.

[8] The same resident may have lived in the home for multiple years and would therefore be present in each calendar year. Most nursing homes provide both long-term residential and short-term rehabilitative care. According to CMS, the number of nursing home residents declined sharply during the pandemic.

indicators highlighted in our review of relevant literature and during conversations with knowledgeable stakeholders.[9] Then, using each resident's calendar year assessments, we determined the percentage of residents experiencing each selected health indicator.[10] We analyzed the data in the CMS Minimum Data Set as they were reported by nursing homes to CMS. We did not otherwise independently verify the accuracy of the information with these nursing homes. We assessed the reliability of the dataset by checking for missing values and obvious errors, reviewing relevant CMS documents, and reviewing other studies that used these data and identified some limitations of our analysis.[11] Based on this review, we determined the data were sufficiently reliable for the purposes of this reporting objective. We also conducted interviews with officials from a non-generalizable sample of nine selected nursing homes in eight selected states: Arkansas, California, Florida,

---

[9] For example, see M. Levere, P. Rowan, A. Wysocki, "The Adverse Effects of the COVID-19 Pandemic on Nursing Home Resident Well -Being," *JAMDA*, vol. 22, no. 5 (2021): 948-954 and L. Fleisher et al., "Health Care Safety During the Pandemic and Beyond—Building a System That Ensures Resilience," *The New England Journal of Medicine*, vol. 386, no. 7 (2022): 609-611.

[10] The mental health indicators we selected and analyzed included whether, on any assessment in a given calendar year, a resident had any symptoms of depression or took anti-depressant, anti-psychotic, or anti-anxiety medications. The physical health indicators we selected and analyzed included whether, on any assessment in a given calendar year, a resident experienced at least one fall, unexplained weight loss, urinary incontinence ranging from occasionally incontinent to always incontinent, or at least one or more stage 1 or higher unhealed pressure ulcers.

[11] Some studies have found that the Minimum Data Set data reported by nursing homes underreports anti-psychotic use and falls. Therefore, it is possible that our analysis also underreports these health indicators. For examples, see HHS Office of Inspector General, CMS Could Improve the Data It Uses to Monitor Antipsychotic Drugs in Nursing Homes, OEI-07-19-00490 (Washington, D.C.: May 3, 2021) and J. Mintz et al., "Validation of the Minimum Data Set Items on Falls and Injury in Two Long-Stay Facilities," Journal of the American Geriatrics Society, vol. 69, no. 4 (April 2021). Unless the rate of underreporting changed during the pandemic, the analysis of change over time would still likely be broadly valid. In addition, as the pandemic progressed, it is possible that nursing homes had to delay submitting their resident assessments if, for example, they were responding to a COVID-19 outbreak. In March 2020, CMS waived the timeframe requirements for nursing homes to complete and transmit resident assessments in order to allow nursing homes to focus on infection control efforts. However, these timeframes were re-instated by CMS in April 2021. According to CMS, the majority of nursing homes were completing and transmitting their assessments in a timely fashion. This is consistent with our analysis, where we determined that less than 10 percent of nursing home quarterly assessments were delayed in each year of our review. See Centers for Medicare & Medicaid Services,
Updates to Long-Term Care Emergency Regulatory Waivers Issued in Response to COVID-19, QSO-21-17-NH (Baltimore, Md.: April 8, 2021).

Maryland, Michigan, Montana, Rhode Island, and Washington.[12] These states were selected based on three criteria: (1) geographic location; (2) number of nursing home beds; and (3) number of nursing home residents and staff with confirmed positive cases of COVID-19.[13] We then selected nursing homes to obtain variation in factors such as bed count and profit or not-for-profit status. We asked nursing home officials to describe resident mental and physical health during the pandemic. Additionally, we interviewed national associations, including the American Health Care Association and National Consumer Voice for Quality Long-Term Care, about these issues.

To describe whether IPC challenges have persisted in nursing homes during the pandemic, we analyzed CMS data on nursing home deficiencies cited by state surveyors in all 50 states and Washington, D.C., from 2018 through 2021.[14] Using these data, we analyzed the deficiency codes used by state surveyors when a nursing home fails to meet CMS's requirements for IPC. We also used CMS's Quality, Certification, and Oversight Reports website to obtain high -level summary data on the percentage of nursing homes with an overdue standard survey.[15] We assessed the reliability of these datasets by checking for missing values and obvious errors and reviewing relevant CMS documents and determined the data were sufficiently reliable for the purposes of this reporting objective. We also conducted interviews with state survey agency officials and nursing home officials in the non-generalizable sample of eight states described above. We asked interviewees to describe the extent to which IPC challenges persisted in nursing homes and how they have responded.

To examine the IPC actions that CMS and CDC have taken related to nursing homes before and during the pandemic, we reviewed CMS and CDC regulations and guidance. We also interviewed officials at CMS and CDC and officials from state survey agencies and nine nursing homes in the non-generalizable sample of eight states described above, as well as officials from the national associations with knowledge of nursing home issues previously noted. We determined that the control environment component of internal

[12] In Washington State, we interviewed officials from two nursing homes, while in the other states, we interviewed officials from one home in each state.

[13] COVID-19 case rates were for the week ending May 16, 2021.

[14] 2021 was the most recent calendar year available at the time of our analysis. In addition, we used the CMS Care Compare Inspection Date files, which were accessed on March 28, 2022 from https://data.cms.gov/provider-data/dataset/svdt-c123.

[15] CMS's Quality, Certification, and Oversight Reports system is a website that provides summary-level data reports on nursing homes. This system is available at https://qcor.cms.gov and was accessed on April 7, 2022.

control was significant to this objective, along with the underlying principle that management should establish expectations of competence for key roles. We also determined that the risk assessment component of internal control was significant to this objective, along with the underlying principle that management should define objectives clearly to enable the identification of risks and define risk tolerances. Finally, we determined that the information and communication component of internal control was significant to this objective, along with the underlying principle that management should use quality information to achieve the entity's objectives. We assessed CMS's oversight activities implemented leading up to and during the COVID-19 pandemic in the context of these internal control principles, as well as HHS statutory requirements, CMS regulatory requirements for nursing home participation in Medicare and Medicaid programs, and CMS's State Operations Manual, to determine whether these oversight actions were clearly defined and understood to enable nursing homes and state survey agencies to address the risk posed by COVID-19; and whether the agency has access to quality information about whether its oversight actions were achieving their stated objectives.[16]

We conducted this performance audit from April 2021 to September 2022 in accordance with generally accepted government auditing standards.

Those standards require that we plan and perform the audit to obtain sufficient, appropriate evidence to provide a reasonable basis for our findings and conclusions based on our audit objectives. We believe that the evidence obtained provides a reasonable basis for our findings and conclusions based on our audit objectives.

Background

Federal law requires nursing homes to keep residents safe from infectious diseases by establishing and maintaining an IPC program designed to help

---

[16] Federal law establishes minimum requirements nursing homes must meet to participate in the Medicare and Medicaid programs, and designates the HHS Secretary as responsible to ensure that requirements governing the provision of care in nursing homes, and the enforcement of such requirements, are adequate to protect the health, safety, welfare, and rights of residents and promote the effective and efficient use of public moneys. 42 U.S.C. §§ 1395i-3(f)(1),1396r(f)(1); 42 C.F.R. §§ 483.1--483.95 (2021).
GAO, Standards for Internal Control in the Federal Government, GAO-14-704G (Washington, D.C.: Sept. 10, 2014). Internal control is a process effected by an entity's oversight body, management, and other personnel that provides reasonable assurance that the objectives of an entity will be achieved.

prevent the development and transmission of communicable diseases and infections.[17]

Infections in Nursing Homes

Even before COVID-19, nursing home residents were at a high risk for several different types of infections, including respiratory infections, gastroenteritis, skin and soft tissue infections, and urinary tract infections. Nursing home residents can be particularly susceptible to infections because of their advanced age and higher risk of comorbidities.[18] Further, nursing home residents are increasingly requiring more medically complex care and are therefore more susceptible to infection. For example, residents discharged from the hospital back to the nursing home can bring infections into the home. They may also require a high-degree of clinical monitoring in order to identify and prevent infection and to help prevent the spread of resistant pathogens between residents. In addition, while nursing homes create important social opportunities for residents through communal dining and recreational spaces, these shared spaces can increase the transmission risk for infectious diseases, especially viruses causing respiratory or gastrointestinal outbreaks.

The COVID-19 pandemic has led to high rates of infection and death in nursing home residents and staff. Nursing home residents are at increased risk because older adults and those with underlying health conditions have a high mortality rate when infected with the virus, according to CDC.[19] In addition, the congregate nature of nursing homes—with staff caring for multiple residents and residents sharing rooms and other communal spaces—can increase the risk that COVID-19 will enter the home and easily spread.[20] The introduction of COVID-19 vaccines in December 2020 resulted in a sharp decline in nursing home cases and deaths through the first part of 2021;

---

[17] 42 U.S.C. §§ 1395i-3(d)(3)(A), 1396r(d)(3)(A); 42 C.F.R. § 483.80 (2021).

[18] Comorbidity refers to the presence of more than one distinct disease in a person at the same time.

[19] Centers for Disease Control and Prevention, *COVID-19: People Who Live in a Nursing Home or Long-Term Care Facility,* accessed on May 7, 2022, https://www.cdc.gov/coronavirus/2019-ncov/need-extra-precautions/people-in-nursing-homes.html.

[20] According to CDC, COVID-19 is spread in three main ways: (1) breathing in small droplets or particles exhaled by an infected person (2) having these small droplets and particles land on the eyes, nose, or mouth, especially through a cough or a sneeze (3) touching eyes, nose, or mouth with hands that have the virus on them. See Centers for Disease Control and Prevention, *How COVID-19 Spreads,* accessed on April 16, 2022, https://www.cdc.gov/coronavirus/2019-ncov/prevent-getting-sick/how-covid-spreads.html.

however, cases and deaths began to increase again with the emergence of more highly transmissible virus variants during the summer of 2021, coinciding with the emergence of the Delta variant, and again in winter 2022, coinciding with the emergence of the Omicron variant.

Federal Oversight of Nursing Homes

Federal laws establish minimum requirements nursing homes must meet to participate in the Medicare and Medicaid programs, including standards for the quality of care.[21] Primarily through its State Operations Manual, CMS establishes the responsibilities of state survey agencies in ensuring that these federal quality standards for nursing homes are met, such as that nursing homes establish and maintain an IPC program.[22] To monitor compliance with these standards, CMS enters into agreements with state survey agencies in each state to assess whether nursing homes meet CMS's standards. Prior to the pandemic, state surveyors from the state survey agencies were responsible for assessing nursing homes using (1) recurring comprehensive standard surveys, or (2) as-needed investigations for complaints from the public and facility-reported incidents.

- Standard surveys. State survey agencies are required by federal law to perform unannounced, on-site standard surveys of every nursing home receiving Medicare or Medicaid payment at least every 15 months, with a statewide average frequency of every 12 months.[23] Standard surveys are important for protecting nursing home residents because they serve as a comprehensive assessment of the safety and quality of nursing home care across several areas including food and

[21] 42 U.S.C. §§ 1395i-3, 1396r; 42 C.F.R. §§ 483.1--483.95 (2021). Federal statutes and their implementing regulations use the terms "skilled nursing facility" (Medicare) and "nursing facility" (Medicaid). For the purposes of this report, we use the term nursing home to refer to both skilled nursing facilities and nursing facilities.

[22] At a minimum, nursing homes must (1) have a system to prevent, identify, report, investigate, and control infections and communicable diseases for all residents, staff, volunteers, visitors, and others providing services in the home; (2) have written standards, policies, and procedures for their infection prevention and control program; (3) have antibiotic use protocols and a system to monitor antibiotic use; and (4) have a system for recording incidents identified under the home's infection prevention and control program and any corrective actions taken. 42 C.F.R. § 483.80(a)(1)-(4) (2021).

[23] 42 U.S.C. §§ 1395i-3(g)(1)(A), (g)(2)(A)(iii), 1396r(g)(1)(A), (g)(2)(A)(iii); 42 C.F.R. §488.308(a)-(b) (2021).

nutrition, resident rights, physician and nursing services, and the physical environment.

- Investigations. In addition to performing standard surveys, state survey agencies are required by federal law to investigate all complaints of nursing home violations of requirements.[24] These fall into two categories: (1) complaints submitted by residents, family members, friends, physicians, and nursing home staff; and (2) "facility-reported incidents" that are self-reported by the nursing homes. These investigations offer the state survey agency a unique opportunity to identify and correct care problems, as they can provide a timely alert of acute issues that otherwise might not be addressed until a standard survey takes place.

If a surveyor from a state survey agency determines that a nursing home violated a federal standard during a survey or investigation, the nursing home is cited for the deficiency using a specific deficiency code (referred to as an F-tag). Cited deficiencies are then classified into categories according to scope (the number of residents potentially affected) and severity (the potential for or occurrence of harm to residents). For most cited deficiencies, nursing homes are required to submit a plan of correction that addresses how the home plans to correct the noncompliance and implement systemic change to ensure the deficient practice would not recur.[25] In addition, when nursing homes are cited with deficiencies, federal enforcement actions can be implemented to encourage homes to make corrections.[26] In general, for deficiencies with a higher scope and severity, CMS may implement the enforcement action immediately.[27] For other deficiencies with a lower scope and severity, the nursing home may be given an opportunity to correct the deficiencies, which, if corrected before the scheduled effective date, can result in the planned enforcement action not being implemented.

---

[24] 42 U.S.C. §§ 1395i-3(g)(4), 1396r(g)(4); 42 C.F.R. § 488.332(a) (2021).

[25] The plan of correction serves as the nursing home's allegation of compliance. Depending on the severity of the deficiency cited, surveyors revisit the nursing home to ensure that the home actually implemented its plan and corrected the deficiency.

[26] CMS does not require enforcement actions be implemented for all deficiencies. Enforcement actions include, but are not limited to, directed in-service training, fines known as civil money penalties, denial of payment, and termination from the Medicare and Medicaid programs.

[27] The scope and severity of a deficiency is one of the factors that CMS may take into account when implementing enforcement actions. CMS may also consider a nursing home's prior compliance history, desired corrective action and long-term compliance, and the number and severity of all the nursing home's deficiencies.

In 2016, CMS finalized a comprehensive update to its nursing home standards.[28] The update included new requirements and aligned existingrequirements with current clinical practices. These standards covered a variety of categories, such as quality of care and IPC.

Prior GAO Work

We have issued several reports examining COVID-19 in nursing homes, part of our larger bodies of work on nursing home oversight and on the federal response to the COVID-19 pandemic (see app. I.) For example, in May 2020, we analyzed CMS deficiency data and found that most nursing homes were cited for IPC deficiencies, such as failure to use proper hand hygiene, in the years prior to the COVID-19 pandemic.[29] In addition, during the COVID-19 pandemic, most nursing homes had multiple outbreaks and weeks of sustained COVID-19 transmission from May 2020 through January 2021.[30] In response to the CARES Act, we have examined the federal response to COVID-19 in nursing homes in multiple reports, where we reported on nursing home-related actions HHS had taken in response to the pandemic, as well as challenges nursing homes faced responding to COVID-19.

Some Indicators of Resident Mental and Physical Health Worsened during the COVID-19 Pandemic

Our analysis of CMS data shows that seven of the eight key indicators of nursing home resident mental and physical health that we reviewed worsened at least slightly in 2020, the first year of the pandemic, compared to the years prior to the pandemic.[31] Six of these key indicators continued to be worse in

[28] Medicare and Medicaid Programs; Reform of Requirements for Long-Term Care Facilities, 81 Fed. Reg. 68,688 (Oct. 4, 2016). Phase 1 (effective November 28, 2016) implemented most minor modifications to the existing nursing home regulations; phase 2 (effective November 28, 2017) implemented new regulations and re-structured CMS's deficiency code system; and phase 3 (effective November 28, 2019) implemented the remaining requirements.

[29] See GAO-20-576R.

[30] 30GAO, COVID-19 in Nursing Homes: Most Homes Had Multiple Outbreaks and Weeks of Sustained Transmission from May 2020 through January 2021, GAO-21-367 (Washington, D.C.: May 19, 2021).

[31] During the COVID-19 pandemic, there have been concerns about mental health in the general population. For example, in January 2021, four in 10 U.S. adults reported symptoms of

the second year of the pandemic than in the years prior to the pandemic.[32] For example, the percentage of residents who experienced depression was 58.7 percent in 2018, 63.9 percent in 2020, and 61.5 percent in 2021. Similarly, the percentage of residents who experienced unexplained weight loss was 14.8 percent in 2018, 19.3 percent in 2020, and 17.4 percent in 2021. (See Figures 1 and 2.)

The results of our data analysis were supported by our interviews with nursing home officials in selected states, who told us they observed worsening resident mental and physical health during the COVID-19 pandemic. Specifically, for resident mental health, officials from some nursing homes we interviewed told us they observed more residents who experienced depression, as well as more residents who took anti-psychotic medication. Nursing home officials and national organizations we interviewed attributed this in part to the isolation residents felt from the limitations CMS placed on visitation or group activities in nursing homes during the pandemic to limit the transmission of COVID-19. CMS initially restricted visitation and suspended group activities in March 2020. After the initial restrictions, CMS made changes to its guidance multiple times during the pandemic to allow for more visitation and group activities, while identifying some situations where limitations would be appropriate to help prevent COVID-19 infections. In November 2021, all visitation limitations were fully lifted.[33]

---

anxiety or depressive disorder, up from one in 10 in 2019. See N. Panchal, R. Kamal, C. Cox, and R. Garfield, *The Implications of COVID-19 for Mental Health and Substance Abuse* (San Francisco, Calif.: Henry J. Kaiser Family Foundation, 2021).

[32] We observed a large decrease (44 percent) in the number of long-stay nursing home residents between 2018 and 2021 (from about 1.9 million to 1.0 million). CMS officials indicated that they also observed a sharp decline in the number of nursing home residents during the pandemic. It is likely that more residents left nursing homes or passed away during the pandemic, either due to COVID-19 or other factors, compared to prior years. It is unclear whether the residents who remained in nursing homes during the pandemic in 2020 and 2021 had different health issues than residents who lived in nursing homes prior to the pandemic.

[33] These restrictions began in March 2020, were changed in September 2020, March 2021, and April 2021, and were fully lifted for all residents in November 2021. See Centers for Medicare & Medicaid Services, *Guidance for Infection Control and Prevention of COVID-19 in Nursing Homes*, QSO-20-14-NH (Baltimore, Md.: March 13, 2020) and Centers for Medicare & Medicaid Services, *Nursing Home Visitation – COVID-19*, QSO-20-39-NH (Baltimore, Md.: Sept. 17, 2020), revised March 10, 2021, April 27, 2021, and November 12, 2021. CMS also released question and answer documents to help enable visitation and frequently asked question documents on visitation, such as this example published March 10, 2022: https://www.cms.gov/files/document/nursing-home-visitation-faq-1223.pdf accessed June 8, 2022.

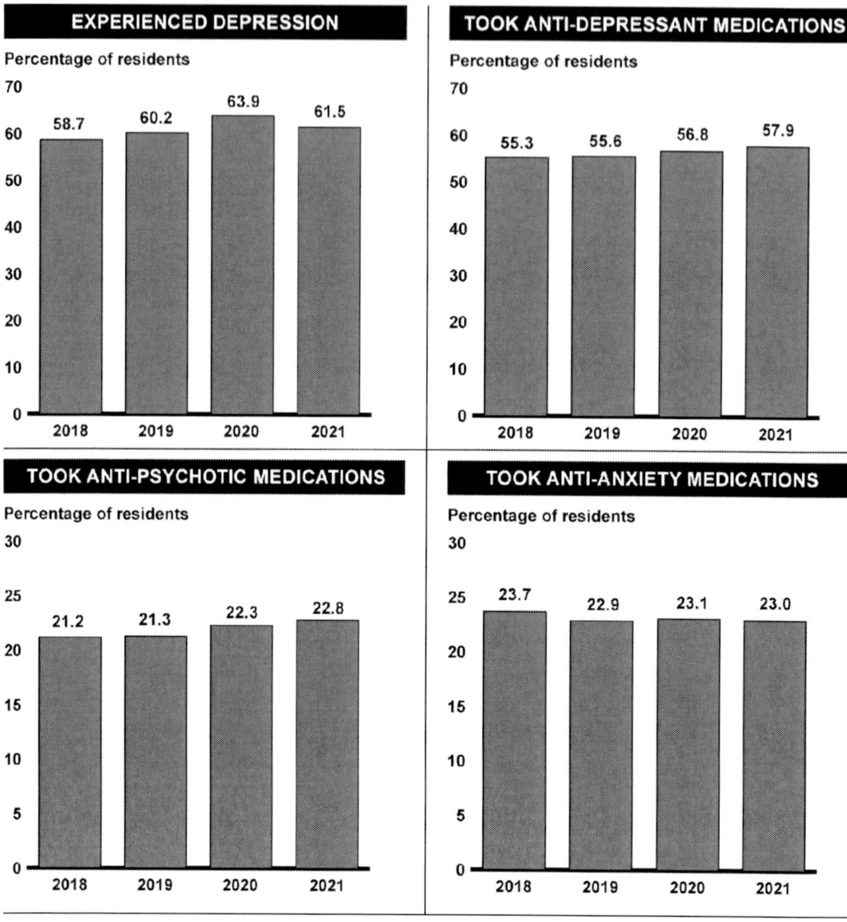

Source: GAO analysis of Centers for Medicare and Medicaid Services (CMS) data. | GAO-22-105133.

Notes: Long-stay residents are those living in a nursing home for greater than 100 days. The data in the Minimum Data Set are self-reported to CMS by nursing homes. "Experienced depression" indicates whether a resident had any symptoms of depression on any assessment in a given calendar year. "Took anti-depressant medications," "took anti-psychotic medications," and "took anti-anxiety medications" indicates if, on any assessment in a given calendar year, a resident took anti-depressant, anti-psychotic, or anti-anxiety medications in the prior 7 days before the assessment or, if less than 7 days, since admission.

Figure 1. Percentage of long-stay nursing home residents who experienced selected mental health indicators, by year.

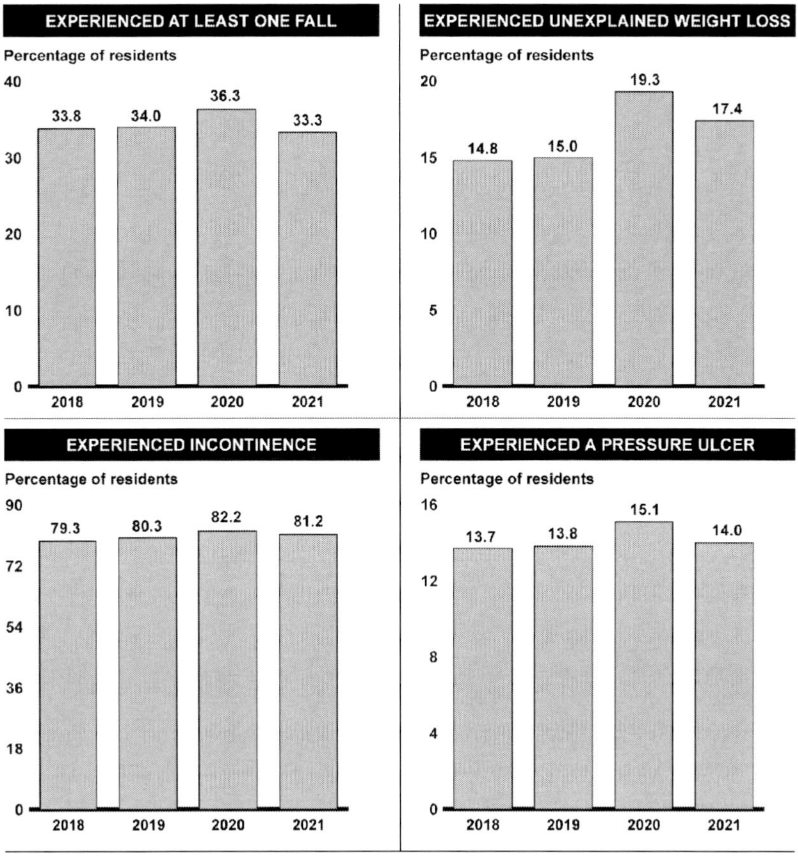

Source: GAO analysis of Centers for Medicare and Medicaid Services (CMS) data. | GAO-22-105133.

Notes: Long-stay residents are those living in a nursing home for greater than 100 days. The data in the Minimum Data Set are self reported to CMS by nursing homes. "Experienced at least one fall" indicates if, on any assessment in a given calendar year, a resident experienced at least one fall since the prior assessment or since admission, whichever was more recent. "Experienced unexplained weight loss" indicates if, on any assessment in a given calendar year, a resident experienced weight loss of 5 percent or more in the last month or 10 percent or more in the last six months. "Experienced incontinence" indicates if, on any assessment in a given calendar year, a resident experienced urinary incontinence ranging from occasionally incontinent to always incontinent. "Experienced at least one pressure ulcer" indicates if, on any assessment in a given calendar year, a resident had at least one or more stage 1 or higher unhealed pressure ulcers.

Figure 2. Percentage of long-stay nursing home residents who experienced selected physical health indicators, by year.

According to CDC, these restrictions were intended to help limit transmission of COVID-19 early in the pandemic, when nursing homes faced multiple complex challenges, including: understanding a novel virus, inability to test to detect asymptomatic infected individuals, variable personal protective equipment supply access, staffing shortages that made controlled visitation more difficult, increasing cases across the country with few effective treatments available, and no vaccine availability.

Nursing home officials in our selected states also told us that they observed worsening resident physical health during the COVID-19 pandemic. Officials from some of the nursing homes we interviewed told us they observed more residents who experienced weight loss and falls when visitation and group activities were limited. One factor contributing to unintended weight loss by residents may have been that, prior to the pandemic, visitors assisted some residents with eating. Officials from one nursing home said that these residents did not eat as well when being fed by a busy staff member rather than an attentive visitor and thus lost weight. Officials from another nursing home said that residents were at a higher risk for falls for various reasons including, for example, they were alone in their rooms and would try to move independently without staff assistance or with inadequate staff assistance. According to CMS, some nursing homes may have been overly restrictive on visitation in a manner that was inconsistent with CMS guidance. CMS noted that the agency requires nursing homes to implement care plans for each resident to attain or maintain the resident's highest practicable physical, mental, and psychosocial well-being.

In November 2021, CMS updated its guidance to allow visitation and group activities with no restrictions, noting that the agency recognized that physical separation from family had taken a physical and emotional toll on residents.[34] Officials from some of the nursing homes we interviewed described seeing a visible improvement in residents once visitation and group activities were allowed again. For example, officials from one selected nursing home said that depression decreased and residents began eating better.

There may be other factors that have contributed to worsening resident mental and physical health during the pandemic. For example, in April 2022, CMS cited significant concerns with the quality of resident care identified by surveyors, such as weight loss, depression, and pressure ulcers as a key rationale for its plans to end certain emergency blanket waivers issued during

---

[34] See Centers for Medicare & Medicaid Services, QSO-20-39-NH (November 12, 2021 revision).

the pandemic, such as waived training requirements for certified nurse aides.[35] In addition, according to one study we reviewed, changes in nursing home resident well-being could be the result of a variety of causes, including the direct effects of being sick with COVID-19, fears associated with contracting the virus, grief from losing friends and loved ones, changes in care practices, such as the declines in the provision of therapy, and other policies put in place to limit the spread of the virus.[36]

Infection Prevention and Control Deficiencies Persisted in Nursing Homes during the COVID-19 Pandemic

The percentage of nursing homes cited for infection prevention and control deficiencies during the COVID-19 pandemic was generally consistent with the years prior. Nursing homes received IPC deficiencies during the COVID-19 pandemic in 2020 and 2021 for failing to follow basic practices, such as proper handwashing, but also for failing to follow COVID-19-specific practices. Officials from the state survey agencies we interviewed said the most persistent IPC challenges in nursing homes during the pandemic were often attributed to staffing challenges. Despite these challenges, stakeholders we interviewed said that nursing homes had gained valuable knowledge about IPC during the pandemic.

The Percentage of Nursing Homes Cited for Infection Prevention and Control Deficiencies During the Pandemic Was Generally Consistent with Prior Years

Our analysis of CMS data shows that the percentage of nursing homes cited for infection prevention and control deficiencies in 2020 and 2021 was

---

[35] CMS noted that by waiving these training requirements, certified nurse aides may not have received the necessary training to, for example, help identify and prevent weight loss in residents. As a result, CMS stated that the agency is concerned about how residents' health and safety has been impacted by the regulations that have been waived. See Centers for Medicare & Medicaid Services, *Update to COVID-19 Emergency Declaration Blanket Waivers for Specific Providers*, QSO-22-15-NH (Baltimore, Md.: April 7, 2022).

[36] See M. Levere, P. Rowan, A. Wysocki, "The Adverse Effects of the COVID-19 Pandemic on Nursing Home Resident Well-Being," *JAMDA*, vol. 22, no. 5 (2021): 948-954.

generally consistent with the years prior.[37] Specifically, about 44 percent of nursing homes were cited for at least one IPC deficiency in 2020, which decreased to about 37 percent in 2021. Prior to the pandemic, in 2018 and 2019, about 43 percent of nursing homes were cited for at least one IPC deficiency. We also previously reported that, in each year from 2013 through 2017, the percent of all nursing homes inspected by state surveyors with an IPC deficiency ranged from 39 to 41 percent.[38]

According to most of the state survey agency officials we interviewed and our review of IPC deficiency narratives written by state surveyors, nursing homes received IPC deficiencies during the pandemic for failing to follow basic IPC practices, such as proper handwashing and personal protective equipment usage, but some state survey officials noted that nursing homes also received IPC deficiencies for failing to follow COVID-19-specific practices such as failing to quarantine and isolate COVID-19 positive residents. (See app. II for illustrative examples of IPC deficiencies.) When examining the severity of the deficiencies cited, we found that in 2018 and 2019, only 1 percent of IPC deficiencies were classified at a high severity where the surveyor determined that residents were harmed or in immediate jeopardy of being harmed.[39] However, during the pandemic in 2020 and 2021, this increased to about 8 and 4 percent, respectively.

CMS put greater emphasis on IPC when it temporarily suspended standard surveys and introduced focused infection control surveys beginning in March 2020. (See app. III for more information on the focused infection control survey and the next finding for how it fits in with other actions CMS took during the pandemic.) While the enhanced scrutiny of IPC through CMS's focused infection control survey does not appear to have resulted in a greater percentage of nursing homes being cited by surveyors for IPC deficiencies

---

[37] For this analysis, we analyzed the deficiency code F-880 for nursing homes that were cited for not meeting federal standards for establishing and maintaining an IPC program.

[38] See GAO-20-576R.

[39] This is consistent with our prior reporting, where we found that, in each year from 2013 through 2017, nearly all IPC deficiencies (about 99 percent in each year) were classified by surveyors as not severe, meaning the surveyor determined that residents were not harmed. See GAO-20-576R.

IPC deficiencies were also categorized by scope—whether the incident was an isolated occurrence, a part of a pattern of behavior, or a widespread behavior. In 2018 and 2019, about 50 percent of IPC deficiencies cited were categorized as isolated, about 30 percent categorized as a pattern, and about 14 percent categorized as widespread. In 2020 and 2021, about 35 percent of IPC deficiencies cited were categorized as isolated, about 40 percent were categorized as pattern, and about 20 percent were categorized as widespread. Percentages do not add to 100 due to rounding.

during the pandemic compared to prior years, the focused infection control surveys were the key source of IPC deficiencies in 2020.[40]

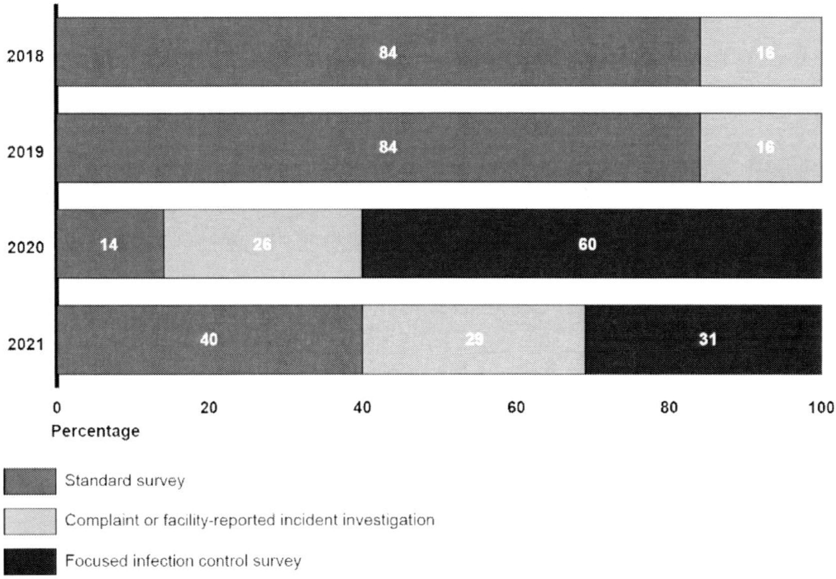

Source: GAO analysis of Centers for Medicare and Medicaid Services (CMS) data. | GAO-22-105133.

Notes: For 352 of the 34,522 IPC deficiencies cited from 2018 through 2021 (about 1 percent), we were unable to determine from CMS's data whether the deficiency was identified during a standard survey, complaint or facility-reported incident investigation, or focused infection control survey. We excluded these deficiencies from our percentages.

Figure 3. Type of survey or investigation used by state survey agencies to identify infection prevention and control deficiencies, 2018 through 2021

---

[40] In January 2021 and again in November 2021, CMS gave state survey agencies more capacity to conduct additional standard surveys by changing the criteria for how often a focused infection control survey must be conducted, after a year of state survey agencies mainly conducting the more frequent focused infection control surveys. See Centers for Medicare & Medicaid Services, *COVID-19 Survey Activities, CARES Act Funding, Enhanced Enforcement for Infection Control Deficiencies, and Quality Improvement Activities in Nursing Homes*, QSO-20-31-ALL (Baltimore, Md.: June 1, 2020) (revised January 4, 2021) and Centers for Medicare & Medicaid Services, *Changes to COVID-19 Survey Activities and Increased Oversight in Nursing Homes*, QSO-22-02-ALL (Baltimore, Md.: Nov. 12, 2021). Nursing homes could be inspected multiple times in a calendar year with a focused infection control survey, depending on the number of outbreaks. On average, nursing homes had four focused infection control surveys in 2020 and three in 2021. In each year from 2018 through 2021, nursing homes had, on average, two complaint or facility-reported incident investigations and one standard survey.

Specifically, our analysis of the CMS data showed that, prior to the pandemic, the vast majority of IPC deficiencies were identified during standard surveys (about 84 percent in 2018 and 2019).[41] In contrast, in 2020, which encompasses the period when standard surveys were temporarily suspended, the majority of IPC deficiencies were identified during focused infection control surveys—60 percent in 2020, which decreased to 31 percent in 2021. Further, as the percentage of IPC deficiencies identified during standard surveys dropped during the pandemic, the percentage of IPC deficiencies identified during complaint or facility-reported incident inspections increased from about 16 percent in 2018 and 2019, to 26 percent in 2020 and 29 percent in 2021. (See Figure 3.)

CMS's suspension of standard surveys and shift to prioritizing the new focused infection control survey in 2020 was a factor contributing to standard survey backlogs in some states due to the growing number of nursing homes exceeding the federal standard of 15 months without a standard survey.[42] According to CMS data, as of April 2022, about 40 percent of nursing homes went at least 16 months without receiving a standard survey.[43] Our review of CMS data found that about 95 percent of nursing homes had a standard survey conducted in each of the 2 years we examined prior to the pandemic. During the pandemic, only 28 percent of nursing homes had a standard survey in 2020 while nearly all homes had at least one focused infection control survey, resulting in half as many total deficiencies as prior to the pandemic. In 2021,

---

[41] For 352 of the 34,522 IPC deficiencies cited from 2018 through 2021 (about 1 percent), we were unable to determine from CMS's data whether the deficiency was identified during a standard survey, complaint or facility-reported incident investigation, or focused infection control survey. We excluded these deficiencies from our percentages.

[42] According to CMS, some state survey agencies had staffing issues during the pandemic that hindered their ability to conduct standard surveys, including staff reassignments and retirements, which also contributed to the backlog. For example, CMS officials said that many states had to pull their surveyors, most of whom were nurses, from their survey roles and deploy them to provide direct care to community residents or to fill other clinical roles in response to the pandemic. Also, many state survey agencies saw an increase in complaint allegations that needed to be investigated, which took resources away from conducting standard surveys.

[43] This is a decrease from May 2021, when the HHS Office of Inspector General reported that 71 percent of nursing homes had gone at least 16 months without receiving a standard survey. See HHS Office of Inspector General, *States' Backlogs of Standard Surveys of Nursing Homes Grew Substantially During the COVID-19 Pandemic*, OEI-01-20-00431 (Washington, D.C.: July 27, 2021). One factor contributing to this decrease could be the steps CMS announced in November 2021 to assist state survey agencies in addressing the backlog of standard surveys, such as by revising the criteria for conducting a focused infection control survey and guidance for resuming standard surveys. See Centers for Medicare & Medicaid Services, QSO-22-02-ALL (Nov. 12, 2021).

about 57 percent of nursing homes had a standard survey, and about 80 percent of nursing homes had at least one focused infection control survey, but the resulting number of total deficiencies cited by surveyors was still about one-quarter less than pre -pandemic levels.[44] This may be because the standard survey provides a comprehensive assessment across multiple areas of a nursing home's safety and quality of care, while the focused infection control survey is more narrowly scoped to assess a nursing home's IPC practices in light of COVID-19.

Our analysis of CMS data shows that a smaller percentage of nursing homes were cited for eight other IPC deficiency codes during the time period examined.[45]_Specifically, four of these eight IPC deficiency codes were established by CMS during the pandemic.[46]_For example, a deficiency code for not meeting federal standards for informing residents, representatives, and families of COVID-19 cases in a nursing home went into effect in May 2020 and, in 2020 and 2021, less than 3 percent of nursing homes inspected by surveyors were cited for this deficiency code.

The remaining four IPC deficiency codes were established by CMS in the years prior to the pandemic. For example, the antibiotic stewardship program deficiency code went into effect in November 2017 and, from 2018 through 2021, 5 percent or less of the nursing homes inspected by surveyors were cited for this deficiency code. (See app. IV for additional data on deficiencies cited.)

Selected State Officials Attributed Persistent Infection Prevention and Control Challenges to Staffing Shortages and High Turnover

Officials from seven of the eight state survey agencies we spoke to said that persistent IPC challenges faced by nursing homes during the pandemic, were rooted in staffing challenges, including staffing shortages and high rates of

---

[44] The percentage of nursing homes with a complaint or facility-reported incident investigation was about 53 percent in 2018, about 56 percent in 2019, about 45 percent in 2020, and about 52 percent in 2021.

[45] These eight other deficiency codes are F-881 for the antibiotic stewardship program, F-882 for the infection preventionist role, F-883 for influenza and pneumococcal immunization, F-945 for infection control training, F-884 for reporting to the National Healthcare Safety Network, F-885 for reporting to residents, representatives, and family, F-886 for COVID-19 testing for residents and staff, and F-887 for COVID-19 immunizations.

[46] See 42 C.F.R. § 483.80(d)(3), (g), (h) (2021).

staff turnover.[47] According to CMS officials, the reasons for staffing shortages can be complex and unclear, ranging from an inadequate recruitment pool to management decisions. Officials we interviewed from four state survey agencies said that, if a nursing home does not have enough staff, it could be challenging for staff to adhere to proper IPC practices, such as taking the time to properly put on and remove personal protective equipment or wash their hands between caring for multiple residents. Officials from one state survey agency we interviewed said that staffing shortages have occurred in nursing homes throughout the pandemic because, for example, employees are out sick.

In addition, officials from four nursing homes we interviewed said that they have sought to adhere to CDC guidance recommending a dedicated space in the home, if possible, for residents with confirmed COVID-19 infections, which has resulted in additional staffing needs.[48] Officials from seven of the nine nursing homes we spoke with said they have experienced a staffing shortage during the pandemic.

Officials from five of the state survey agencies we spoke with noted that there had been a lot of staff turnover during the pandemic, which made it difficult for a home to ensure that new or temporary staff are trained on IPC. (In response to the pandemic, CMS gave nursing homes more flexibility in hiring temporary employees to work as nurse aides by suspending certain training and certification requirements.[49]) According to officials from one state survey agency, some of these temporary employees had never worked in a nursing home before. Officials from some nursing homes we interviewed also reported using temporary staff from nurse staffing agencies. Officials we interviewed from three state survey agencies said that while nursing homes typically do in -service training for their own permanent staff, they may not

---

[47] Even before the COVID-19 pandemic, nursing homes have historically struggled with staffing shortages and high rates of staff turnover. For more, see National Academies of Sciences, Engineering, and Medicine, *The National Imperative to Improve Nursing Home Quality: Honoring Our Commitment to Nursing Home Residents, Families, and Staff* (Washington, D.C.: The National Academies Press, 2022).

[48] CDC guidance specifies that staff should be assigned to work only in this unit when it is in use and that at a minimum, staff in the COVID-19 unit should include the primary nursing assistants and nurses assigned to care for these residents. Accessed on November 8, 2021, https://www.cdc.gov/coronavirus/2019-ncov/hcp/long-term-care.html.

[49] Specifically, from March 2020 through June 2022, CMS waived the requirement that a nursing home not employ anyone for more than 4 months unless they meet certain training and certification requirements to address potential staffing shortages in nursing homes due to the COVID-19 pandemic. See Centers for Medicare & Medicaid Services, COVID-19 Emergency Declaration Blanket Waivers for Health Care Providers, (Baltimore, Md.: March 13, 2020) and Centers for Medicare & Medicaid Services, QSO-22-15-NH (April 7, 2022).

have had the time or resources to provide the same training to temporary staff during the pandemic, including staff from nurse staffing agencies. Officials from seven nursing homes we interviewed noted that this was compounded by the challenges of keeping staff trained on guidance, which officials said was constantly changing due to the changing circumstances of the pandemic.

Despite Challenges, Nursing Home Officials from Selected States Reported Gaining Knowledge About Infection Prevention and Control Practices During the Pandemic

Nursing home officials we interviewed from our selected states said that nursing homes gained valuable knowledge about IPC practices during the COVID-19 pandemic. For example, nursing home officials said their understanding of the significance and additional application of basic IPC practices—such as the importance of proper handwashing and the proper use of personal protective equipment—was enhanced. Officials from one nursing home said that, prior to the pandemic, the home would conduct an annual IPC "boot camp" training but the pandemic taught them that those IPC skills were easy to forget when they were not constantly put into practice. An official from another nursing home said that the IPC lessons that staff learned during the COVID-19 pandemic were applicable to preventing the spread of other types of infections.

Nursing home officials, we interviewed also described learning new COVID-19 specific practices, such as how to conduct on-site testing, set up quarantine and isolation units, and screen visitors and staff. Officials from one nursing home described developing a process for swabbing and testing nearly 150 staff members for COVID-19 twice a week. Officials from another nursing home said they learned how to work with the design of their building to locate adequate quarantine and isolation spaces. Officials from two other nursing homes described IPC practices they implemented during the pandemic that they hoped to continue going forward. For example, officials from one nursing home said that when the pandemic ends they plan to continue the visitor and staff symptom screening they put in place for COVID-19 to prevent the spread of infections.

CMS and CDC Took Actions to Strengthen Infection Prevention and Control but Should Do More

CMS and CDC Took Numerous Actions on Infection Prevention and Control

Our review of agency documentation and interviews with agency officials show that CMS and CDC took numerous actions to improve infection prevention and control both prior to and during the pandemic. For example, prior to the pandemic, CMS required nursing homes to designate an infection preventionist on staff and, during the pandemic, CMS and CDC provided infection prevention resources to nursing homes. (See app. V for a full list of IPC actions identified by CMS and CDC.)

The infection preventionist role

The infection preventionist is a nursing home employee with training in infection prevention and control who is responsible for the home's program for preventing, identifying, reporting, investigating, and controlling infections and communicable diseases. Beginning November 2019, the Centers for Medicare & Medicaid Services (CMS) required all nursing homes to designate one or more infection preventionists who has completed specialized training in infection prevention and control and who works at the nursing home at least part-time. Some of the responsibilities of the infection preventionist may include contact tracing during an infectious disease outbreak, reporting surveillance data, and educating staff on proper adherence to infection prevention and control practices.

Source: GAO summary of CMS and the Centers for Disease Control and Prevention documents. | GAO-22-105133.

Examples of actions CMS and CDC took prior to the COVID-19 pandemic include the following:

- *Required designated infection preventionist.* CMS updated IPC requirements to include the requirement that nursing homes designate at least one infection preventionist to oversee the facility's IPC program, effective beginning November 2019.

- *Developed infection preventionist training.* To support the infection preventionist requirement, CMS, in consultation with CDC, developed a free online infection preventionist training program that was available to nursing homes as of March 2019.[50] The specialized training provided content covering a range of IPC topics to prepare infection preventionists for their role.
- *Conducted IPC pilot program and released Infection Control Worksheet tool.* To help assess and prevent infections in nursing homes, CMS, in consultation with CDC, conducted a 3-year IPC pilot project from fiscal year 2016 through 2018, which used a worksheet tool, developed with CDC and expert input, to identify gaps in nursing home IPC practices and guide assistance to address those gaps.[51] CMS released the worksheet as an IPC self-assessment tool to nursing homes in November 2019.[52]

Examples of key actions CMS and CDC took during the pandemic include the following:

- *Initiated focused infection control surveys.* In March 2020, CMS made key changes in how it oversees nursing homes by requiring state survey agencies to conduct a new survey type known as the focused infection control survey that assessed IPC-related requirements specific to COVID-19, such as adherence to visitorscreening and personal protective equipment protocols.[53] (See app. III.)
- *Restricted visitation and group activities.* In March 2020, to limit the transmission of COVID-19, CMS temporarily restricted visitation from all visitors and non-essential health care personnel, except for

---

[50] See Centers for Medicare & Medicaid Services, Specialized Infection Prevention and Control Training for Nursing Home Staff in the Long-Term Care Setting is Now Available, QSO-19-10-NH (Baltimore, Md.: March 11, 2019).

[51] See Centers for Medicare & Medicaid Services, Infection Control Pilot Project, S&C-16-05-ALL (Baltimore, Md.: Dec. 23, 2015).

[52] For the pilot, the new survey tool was used for educational purposes rather than to assess compliance with existing IPC requirements. After the surveyors assessed the participating nursing homes' IPC practices, the nursing homes were provided with technical assistance based on the survey's results. See Centers for Medicare & Medicaid Services, S&C-16-05-ALL (Dec. 23, 2015).

[53] CMS continued to require state survey agencies to conduct high-priority complaint investigations, such as those conducted in response to alleged abuse or neglect. See Centers for Medicare & Medicaid Services, Prioritization of Survey Activities, QSO-20-20-ALL (Baltimore, Md.: March 20, 2020).

certain compassionate care situations and suspended group activities.[54] In November 2021, CMS lifted these restrictions.[55]

- *Developed IPC-specific training and technical assistance.* CMS and CDC developed training and technical assistance resources to help nursing homes implement IPC practices. For example, in May 2020, CMS released a toolkit of COVID-19 best practices.[56] In June 2020, CMS deployed a network of quality improvement organizations to provide technical assistance to approximately 3,000 low performing nursing homes with a history of infection control challenges.[57] Beginning in July 2020, CDC deployed "strike teams" of infection prevention and public health professionals to nursing homes facing challenges with infection control.[58] In August 2020, CMS released online IPC training courses developed in consultation with CDC.
- *Mandated COVID-19 surveillance reporting.* In May 2020, CMS required nursing homes to report data at least weekly through CDC's National Healthcare Safety Network on COVID-19 cases and deaths among residents and staff, personal protective equipment supplies, access to testing, and staff shortages, among other things.[59]

---

[54] These restrictions included ombudsmen, which are advocates for nursing home residents. These restrictions were later clarified to allow certain conditions for visitation, such as to allow residents access to long-term care ombudsmen. See Centers for Medicare & Medicaid Services, QSO-20-14-NH (Mar. 13, 2020 revision) and Centers for Medicare & Medicaid Services, Nursing Home Five Star Quality Rating System Updates, Nursing Home Staff Counts, Frequently Asked Questions, and Access to Ombudsman, QSO-20-28-NH (Baltimore, Md.: April 24, 2020 and Jul. 9, 2020 revision). After the initial restrictions, CMS made changes to its visitation guidance multiple times during the pandemic to allow increased visitation and group activities. See Centers for Medicare & Medicaid Services QSO-20-39-NH (Sept. 17, 2020), revised March 10, 2021 and April 27, 2021.

[55] See Centers for Medicare & Medicaid Services, QSO-20-39-NH (Nov. 12, 2021 revision).

[56] See Centers for Medicare & Medicaid Services, *CMS Issues Nursing Homes Best Practices Toolkit to Combat COVID-19*, May 13, 2020, accessed April 18, 2022, https://www.cms.gov/newsroom/press-releases/cms-issues-nursing-homes-best-practices-toolkit-combat-covid-19.

[57] See Centers for Medicare & Medicaid Services, QSO-20-31-ALL (June 1, 2020).

[58] The strike teams identified challenges related to staffing, personal protective equipment supplies, COVID-19 testing, and infection prevention and control measure implementation. See L. Anderson et al., "Protecting Nursing Home Residents from COVID-19: Federal Strike Team Findings and Lessons Learned," *New England Journal of Medicine Catalyst* (June 28, 2021).

[59] 85 Fed. Reg. 27,550, 27,627 (May 8, 2020) (codified at 42 C.F.R. § 483.80(g)). Until December 31, 2024, the new requirement provides for these data to be reported at the federal level through CDC's National Healthcare Safety Network and to be updated and publicly reported. Prior to this reporting requirement, state and local health departments may have required nursing homes to report certain COVID-19 related information to them

- *Increased IPC enforcement actions.* In June 2020, CMS increased financial and other penalties, such as requiring directed plans of correction, for nursing home noncompliance with IPC requirements and made enforcement actions more significant for nursing homes with a history of past infection control deficiencies.[60]

Stakeholders Reported Advantages and Disadvantages of CMS and CDC Infection Prevention and Control Actions

Nursing home and state survey agency officials reported to us what they believed were advantages and disadvantages for selected IPC actions taken before and during the pandemic. For example, state survey agency and nursing home officials told us that CMS's requirement to designate an infection preventionist was crucial to nursing homes during the COVID-19 pandemic. See Table 1.

Table 1. Selected Federal Infection Prevention and Control (IPC) actions and examples of stakeholder-reported perspectives on advantages and disadvantages

Action	Description	Advantages	Disadvantages
Required designated infection preventionist	The Centers for Medicare & Medicaid Services	• Critical role in nursing homes during the pandemic (eight	• Requirement needs strengthening to ensure sufficient

as part of their infectious disease surveillance programs. See 42 C.F.R. § 483.80(a)(2)(ii) (2021). In May 2021, CMS also required nursing homes to report COVID-19 vaccine and therapeutics treatment information to the CDC's National Healthcare Safety Network. Medicare and Medicaid Programs; COVID–19 Vaccine Requirements for Long-Term Care Facilities and Intermediate Care Facilities for Individuals with Intellectual Disabilities Residents, Clients, and Staff, 86 Fed. Reg. 26,306, 26,336 (May 13, 2021) (codified at 42 C.F.R. § 483.80(g)(1)(viii)-(ix)).

[60] As part of these efforts, CMS encouraged state survey agencies to develop and issue to noncompliant nursing homes directed plans of correction, as their enforcement action, in which state survey agencies specify actions a nursing home must take to address infection control deficiencies, such as obtaining further IPC training or hiring an IPC consultant. See Centers for Medicare & Medicaid Services, QSO-20-31-ALL (June 1, 2020). On February 28, 2022, the White House announced that it would lead further efforts to improve quality and safety in nursing homes through enforcement actions. For example, it announced a commitment to hold poorly performing nursing homes accountable for improper and unsafe care by expanding financial penalties and other sanctions and including more nursing homes in an enhanced oversight program targeting the poorest performers.

Table 1. (Continued)

Action	Description	Advantages	Disadvantages
	(CMS) updated IPC requirements to include the designation of infection preventionists.	of nine nursing homes and five of eight state survey agencies)	infection preventionist staffing levels (two of nine nursing homes and three of eight state survey agencies) • Difficult to hire or retain infection prevention professionals in order to comply (one of nine nursing homes and two of eight state survey agencies)
Developed infection preventionist training	CMS, in consultation with the Centers for Disease Control and Prevention (CDC), developed infection preventionist training in preparation for the infection preventionist requirement.	• Training is helpful, comprehensive (six of nine nursing homes and three of eight state survey agencies)	• Training is time intensive (one of nine nursing homes and two of eight state survey agencies) • Training curriculum is limited, other training opportunities needed (one of nine nursing homes and four of eight state survey agencies)
Conducted IPC pilot program and released Infection Control Worksheet	CMS, in consultation with CDC, conducted a pilot from fiscal year 2016 through 2018 to help prevent the spread of infections in nursing homes. CMS released the Infection Control Worksheet for nursing homes.	Generally, the information we gathered from stakeholders indicated limited awareness of the worksheet as a tool to help nursing homes.	

Action	Description	Advantages	Disadvantages
Initiated focused infection control surveys	CMS developed the focused infection control survey to assess IPC-related requirements specific to COVID-19.	• Helps improve IPC practices (seven of nine nursing homes and four of eight state survey agencies)	• Punitive rather than helpful approach (five of nine nursing homes and one of eight state survey agencies) • Frequent and distracting from resident care (four of nine nursing homes and five of eight state survey agencies) • Guidance unclear (three of nine nursing homes and eight of eight state survey agencies) • Contributed to state survey agencies' backlogs of standard surveys (six of eight state survey agencies)
Restricted visitation and suspended group activities	CMS temporarily restricted nursing home visitation and suspended group activities.	• Necessary to keep residents and staff safe (three of nine nursing homes and four of eight state survey agencies)	• Isolated residents and resulted in some mental or physical declines in health (six of nine nursing homes and five of eight state survey agencies)
Developed IPC-specific training and technical assistance	CMS and CDC developed training and technical assistance resources to help nursing homes implement IPC practices.	• Helps improve IPC practices (six of nine nursing homes and six of eight state survey agencies)	• Content basic or not timely and accessible (three of nine nursing homes and six of eight state survey agencies)
Mandated COVID-19 surveillance reporting	CMS required nursing homes to report to CDC weekly surveillance data, such as COVID-19 cases and deaths.	• Useful for directing resources and policy improvements (one of nine nursing homes and four of eight state survey agencies)	• Weekly reporting burden (five of nine nursing homes and four of eight state survey agencies) • Lack of clear training and instructions (three of nine nursing homes)

Table 1. (Continued)

Action	Description	Advantages	Disadvantages
Increased IPC enforcement actions	CMS increased financial and other penalties for nursing home noncompliance with IPC requirements.	• Incentivizes improvements (five of eight state survey agencies) • Provides more effective options, such as directed plans of correction, for system change (four of eight state survey agencies)	• Overly punitive during a pandemic (four of nine nursing homes and five of eight state survey agencies)

Source: GAO interviews with selected state survey agency and nursing home officials in eight states. | GAO-22-105133.

CMS Has Opportunities to Strengthen Infection Prevention and Control Oversight Strengthen Oversight of the Infection Preventionist Role

In our review of CMS IPC oversight, we identified areas where CMS could take more actions to strengthen oversight of IPC in nursing homes. Specifically, we found that CMS could take steps to strengthen both the role of the infection preventionist in nursing homes and IPC guidance.

As previously described, most nursing home and state survey agency officials we interviewed indicated that CMS's requirement that nursing homes have an infection preventionist was critical to helping nursing homes address IPC challenges during the pandemic. Some of these officials, representing two very distinct perspectives, suggested CMS take actions to clarify and strengthen requirements for the role. We identified two ways that CMS could strengthen its oversight of the infection preventionist role: (1) establish minimum training standards and (2) collect and use infection preventionist staffing data to assess the sufficiency of the current staffing requirement.

Establish minimum infection preventionist training standards. We found that training for nursing home infection preventionists is inconsistent because CMS has not specified the minimum training that infection preventionists need to receive so that they can be effective performing their role in nursing homes.

As part of its 2016 regulatory update of nursing home requirements, CMS began requiring nursing homes to designate an infection preventionist by November 28, 2019, and required infection preventionists to have completed "specialized training in IPC." However, the requirement lacks specificity about what, at a minimum, the specialized training should comprise. According to CMS, the agency does not set minimum training requirements for other types of nursing home personnel and expects nursing homes to provide the amount of training needed to ensure staff have the skills to do their jobs.[61] One state survey agency official told us that nursing homes are using a variety of training programs that are not equally rigorous to meet the CMS requirement, each with different curricula and covering different topics. Therefore, the official saw a need for standardizing infection preventionist training programs.[62] Further, survey results from a 2018 study found that only 39 percent of nursing homes surveyed reported that their infection preventionists had completed specialized training in IPC.[63] Additionally, CMS, CDC, and state survey agency officials from some of our selected states identified noticeable gaps in the skills of nursing home infection preventionists during the pandemic, with CMS and CDC officials noting that some infection preventionists were unable to develop strategies for addressing common IPC practice errors, such as with hand hygiene. According to CMS and CDC officials, there are numerous trainings available for infection preventionists, including a comprehensive training program developed by CMS, in consultation with CDC, in March of 2019.

Establishing minimum training requirements would be consistent with federal standards for internal control that call for management to set clear expectations of competence for key roles, such as the role of the infection preventionist.[64] CMS planned to issue additional guidance to clarify the role

---

[61] CMS said that the agency requires nurse aides to complete 75 hours of training, because this minimum initial training standard is established in statute. See 42 U.S.C. §§ 1395i-3(f)(2)(A)(i)(II), 1396r(f)(2)(A)(i)(II).

[62] Further, CDC officials said that historically there have been limited training courses available for a nursing home infection preventionist to obtain nursing-home specific IPC knowledge because many of the available training programs were not initially designed for nursing home settings. CDC officials also noted that since 2016, when the infection preventionist requirement was published, multiple courses have been developed and that these courses may be variable in terms of training time and topics since they were not developed in response to required specifications.
In addition, studies have found a lack of training among the personnel responsible for infection prevention and control in nursing homes. See National Academies of Sciences, Engineering, and Medicine, *The National Imperative to Improve Nursing Home Quality: Honoring Our Commitment to Nursing Home Residents, Families, and Staff* (Washington, D.C.: The National Academies Press, 2022).

[63] P. Stone et al., "Nursing Home Infection Control Program Characteristics, CMS Citations, and Implementation of Antibiotic Stewardship Policies: A National Study," *INQUIRY: The Journal of Health Care Organization, Provision, and Financing*, vol. 55 (2018) 1-7.

[64] GAO-14-704G.

of the infection preventionist, which could include more information about the minimum training infection preventionists need, but CMS officials told us that the agency has delayed issuance multiple times due to the COVID-19 pandemic. In June 2022, CMS released an advance copy of guidance, which clarifies the role of the infection preventionist but does not clarify infection preventionists' minimum training requirements, such as how many hours of training infection preventionists must complete.[65] Until CMS establishes minimum training standards for infection preventionists, nursing homes may not know which training programs are adequate and required for preparing their infection preventionists, and the skills of infection preventionists may not be adequate to allow them to effectively perform their role.

Collect and use infection preventionist staffing data. We found that CMS does not collect staffing data on infection preventionists in its staffing data system as it does for other positions. As a result, the agency lacks information it could use to assess whether CMS's minimum staffing standard for a part-time infection preventionist is sufficient to address infection risks to both residents and staff in all nursing homes.

Some nursing home and state survey agency officials from our selected states told us that many part-time infection preventionists do not have sufficient time to conduct the IPC tasks that could limit the risk of infections. Specifically, we heard from some of the nursing homes and state survey agency officials that having only a part-time infection preventionist was not sufficient for some homes. Infection preventionists we interviewed from five of nine nursing homes in our review were staff members who shared other significant and demanding roles, such as serving as the Director of Nursing, and, as a result, some were hampered in their ability to carry out all of their infection prevention responsibilities. For example, one nursing home infection preventionist said that, because she also serves as the facility's assistant director of nursing, often her infection preventionist role is a "second thought assignment."

When discussing the requirement that nursing homes must have at least one part-time infection preventionist on staff, CMS officials told us the requirement was designed to allow nursing homes flexibility to determine the amount of time needed for an infection preventionist to effectively oversee the facility's IPC program. In June 2022, CMS released an advance copy of guidance, which notes that, while the CMS requirement is to have an infection

[65] See Centers for Medicare & Medicaid Services, Revised Long-Term Care Surveyor Guidance, QSO-22-19-NH (Baltimore, Md.: June 29, 2022).

preventionist at least part-time, nursing homes are responsible for an effective IPC program and should ensure the role of the infection preventionist is tailored to meet the nursing home's needs.[66] However, nursing home and state survey agency officials from four states in our review told us that nursing homes do not always dedicate funding to hire infection preventionists beyond the minimum required, regardless of the need. Finally, the CMS Coronavirus Commission for Safety and Quality in Nursing Homes' report from September 2020, highlighted findings that part-time infection preventionists often cannot adequately respond to the demands of the COVID -19 pandemic and recommended that CMS determine whether or under what circumstances nursing homes should have more than one part-time preventionist.[67]

To the extent that CMS's current infection preventionist requirement may be inadequate for some nursing homes, it poses a potential risk to CMS's goal of ensuring quality care for nursing home residents. Addressing risk is consistent with federal standards for internal control that call for management to identify, analyze, and respond to risks by estimating their effect on achieving a defined objective.[68] CMS could begin to assess this risk with data on preventionist staffing levels across the nursing homes it oversees. It could require nursing homes to submit staffing data on infection preventionists through its Payroll Based Journal System, as it does with other staffing positions, which would result in the agency having comprehensive data on the number of hours infection preventionists are paid to work each day.[69] CMS could then use these staffing data to examine what level of infection preventionist staffing is needed based on nursing home size and the complexity of resident care needs. The agency could also use the data to compare the relationship, if any, between IPC deficiencies and infection preventionist staffing levels. CMS does not currently collect the infection

---

[66] See Centers for Medicare & Medicaid Services, QSO-22-19-NH (June 29, 2022).

[67] Specifically, the commission recommended that CMS establish an evidence-based standard for an infection preventionist educator full-time equivalent to bed ratio, among a number of other recommended steps CMS could take to strengthen the role of infection preventionists in nursing homes. See MITRE, Coronavirus Commission on Safety and Quality in Nursing Homes, *Commission Final Report* (McLean, Va.: The MITRE Corporation, 2020). This report was written for CMS under a government contract.

[68] GAO-14-704G.

[69] The Payroll Based Journal System was developed in 2015 in response to the Patient Protection and Affordable Care Act, which required CMS to establish a national system to collect and report payroll data on nurse staffing hours. Pub. L. No. 111-148, §§ 6103, 6106, 124 Stat. 119, 704 (2010) (codified at 42 U.S.C. §§ 1320-7j(g), 1395i-3(i)(1)(A)(i)), 1396r(i)(1)(A)(i)). The system allows the agency to collect staffing data on a regular and more frequent basis than previously, when the data were reported by the homes during surveys, and the system allows the data to be auditable to ensure accuracy.

preventionist staffing data in this way because the infection preventionist role was created after the Payroll Based Journal System was rolled out in 2015.

Collecting and utilizing quality information to inform agency decisions is consistent with federal standards for internal control to use quality information to achieve objectives.[70] Having comprehensive data on infection preventionist staffing levels across nursing homes would allow the agency to begin assessing whether the standard is sufficient for protecting nursing home residents and staff or whether it needs to be modified.

Strengthen Infection Prevention and Control Guidance

As previously described, some nursing home and state survey agency officials from our selected states indicated that the guidance issued by CMS for some IPC oversight actions was unclear and, in some situations, resulted in concerns about the enforcement actions taken against nursing homes. We identified how CMS could strengthen its guidance around IPC oversight actions by providing additional guidance to help nursing homes and state survey agencies to assess IPC practices.

We found that CMS's State Operations Manual—the key guidance state survey agencies use for conducting nursing home surveys—does not contain important IPC-related guidance. Specifically, as of May 2022, the State Operations Manual does not have examples that surveyors can use to assess the scope and severity of deficiencies applicable to COVID-19-related IPC requirements. For example, the scope and severity examples for the IPC deficiency code (F-880) did not include examples related to the use of personal protective equipment, cohorting (or grouping) residents and staff to limit opportunities for transmission, and quarantining, that may be more applicable to stopping the spread of outbreaks from COVID-19 and other respiratory diseases spread by droplets and aerosols (e.g., influenza).[71] According to

---

[70] GAO-14-704G.

[71] While Appendix PP of the State Operations Manual provides examples of non-compliance with precautions around topics such as bloodborne infections, gastrointestinal illness, and the handling of soiled linens during scabies or head lice outbreaks, the manual does not contain examples of scope and severity categorization for deficiencies related to masking, cohorting and quarantining, or other precautions that may be more applicable to COVID-19 or other respiratory diseases such as influenza transmission. See Centers for Medicare & Medicaid Services, *State Operations Manual, Appendix PP—Guidance to Surveyors for Long Term Care Facilities* (Baltimore, Md.: November 22, 2017). In June 2022, CMS

CMS, routine updates to the State Operations Manual have not been made during the pandemic due to the temporary nature of certain guidance and the need for issuing more frequent, immediate updates, which CMS released through memoranda. In June 2022, while this report was with the agency for review and comment, CMS released an advance copy of the State Operations Manual to provide additional guidance to state surveyors for IPC-related deficiencies, including additional scope and severity classification examples, but these examples were not specific to COVID-or other types of respiratory diseases. Without COVID-19-relevant examples for scope and severity classification, some state survey agencies told us they are sometimes uncertain about how to inspect nursing homes for adherence to COVID-19 specific requirements, which officials say can lead to surveyors applying these requirements inconsistently.

Clarifying its guidance for surveyors would be consistent with CMS's State Operations Manual, which states that CMS is responsible for "conveying operational instructions and official interpretations of policy."[72] It would also be consistent with federal standards for internal control that indicate management should communicate the necessary quality information to achieve its objectives.[73] By providing examples of scope and severity determinations for IPC related issues in the State Operations Manual, CMS can help ensure that state survey agencies are better able to understand and uphold the requirements for managing COVID-19 and other infectious diseases.

Conclusion

The COVID-19 pandemic has not only led to high rates of severe illness and death in the nation's nursing homes, but it also contributed to worsened mental and physical health among residents and highlighted persistent problems with infection prevention and control. While CMS and CDC have taken important actions to try to improve nursing home infection prevention and control both prior to and during the COVID-19 pandemic, there is more CMS should do. First, CMS should do more to strengthen oversight of the role of the infection

---

released an advance copy of Appendix PP that will go into effect on October 24, 2022. See Centers for Medicare & Medicaid Services, QSO-22-19-NH (June 29, 2022).

[72] Centers for Medicare & Medicaid Services, *State Operations Manual, Chapter 1— Program Background and Responsibilities* (Baltimore, Md.: October 3, 2014).

[73] GAO-14-704G.

preventionist, a position whose creation was reported to be critical for helping nursing homes during the pandemic. Specifically, until CMS sets minimum training standards for infection preventionists, nursing homes will not know which training programs are adequate for preparing their infection preventionists, and the skills of infection preventionists may not be adequate to allow them to effectively perform their role. Similarly, until CMS collects and uses infection preventionist staffing data, the agency will lack information critical to understanding whether infection preventionists are dedicating enough time to IPC to meet the risks of infectious disease in nursing homes. Finally, CMS should clarify its IPC guidance to nursing homes and state survey agencies. Specifically, until CMS clarifies guidance on the scope and severity examples for IPC deficiencies specific to COVID-19 and other respiratory diseases, state survey agencies will continue to face uncertainty about how to inspect nursing homes for adherence to IPC requirements.

Recommendations for Executive Action

We are making the following three recommendations to the Administrator of CMS to:

1. Establish minimum infection preventionist training standards. (Recommendation 1)
2. Collect infection preventionist staffing data and use these data to determine whether the current infection preventionist staffing requirement is sufficient. (Recommendation 2)
3. Provide additional guidance in the State Operations Manual on making scope and severity determinations for IPC-related deficiencies. (Recommendation 3)

Agency Comments and Our Evaluation

We provided a draft of this report to HHS for review and comment. In its written comments, printed in appendix VI, HHS agreed with the first of our three recommendations, but did not state whether the department agreed or disagreed with our other two recommendations.

Specifically, HHS concurred with our first recommendation and noted that CMS will consider this recommendation when proposing new requirements through the rulemaking process.

Regarding our second recommendation, while HHS did not specifically state whether it agreed or disagreed, the department said that CMS will consider this recommendation when proposing new requirements through the rulemaking process. Further, HHS said that CMS will evaluate the feasibility of collecting infection preventionist staffing data and take appropriate actions based on this evaluation.

Regarding our third recommendation, HHS did not state whether it agreed or disagreed, but the department noted that it believes that CMS addressed this recommendation prior to GAO's report publication and therefore requested that GAO remove this recommendation. In June 2022, while a draft of this report was with HHS for review and comment, CMS released an advance copy of revised guidance, including revisions to sections of the State Operations Manual relevant to this recommendation. CMS stated that the agency believes this revised guidance addresses this recommendation. In response, we updated our report to reflect this revised guidance. We acknowledge that the revisions, scheduled to go into effect in October 2022 provide needed additional guidance on determining the scope and severity of IPC-related deficiencies. However, none of the revised scope and severity examples relate to stopping the spread of outbreaks from COVID-19 or other respiratory diseases spread by droplets and aerosols (e.g., influenza), as we describe in our report. For example, as we note in our report, none of the examples in the prior guidance or the revised guidance relate to the use of personal protective equipment, cohorting residents and staff, or quarantining residents to limit opportunities for transmission. While we recognize that CMS has taken some important steps toward addressing the clarity of the scope and severity examples in the recent update, we maintain the importance of having examples related to COVID-19 or respiratory diseases more generally in this guidance. In addition, HHS also provided technical comments, which we incorporated as appropriate.

List of Addressees

The Honorable Patrick Leahy
Chairman

The Honorable Richard Shelby
Vice Chairman
Committee on Appropriations
United States Senate

The Honorable Ron Wyden
Chairman

The Honorable Mike Crapo
Ranking Member
Committee on Finance
United States Senate

The Honorable Patty Murray
Chair

The Honorable Richard Burr
Ranking Member
Committee on Health, Education, Labor, and Pensions
United States Senate

The Honorable Gary C. Peters
Chairman

The Honorable Rob Portman
Ranking Member
Committee on Homeland Security and Governmental Affairs
United States Senate

The Honorable Rosa L. DeLauro
Chair

The Honorable Kay Granger
Ranking Member
Committee on Appropriations
House of Representatives

The Honorable Frank Pallone, Jr.
Chairman

The Honorable Cathy McMorris Rodgers
Republican Leader
Committee on Energy and Commerce
House of Representatives

The Honorable Bennie G. Thompson
Chairman

The Honorable John Katko
Ranking Member
Committee on Homeland Security
House of Representatives

The Honorable Carolyn B. Maloney
Chairwoman
The Honorable James Comer
Ranking Member
Committee on Oversight and Reform
House of Representatives

The Honorable Richard E. Neal
Chairman

The Honorable Kevin Brady
Republican Leader
Committee on Ways and Means
House of Representatives

The Honorable Michael F. Bennet
United States Senate

Appendix II: Examples of Infection Prevention and Control Deficiencies Cited in Nursing Homes during the Pandemic

Infection prevention and control (IPC) practices can be critical to preventing the spread of infectious diseases, including those specific to COVID-19. We reviewed examples of IPC deficiency narratives written by state surveyors to illustrate IPC deficiencies from different time points during the pandemic.

Table 2. Illustrative examples of narratives from infection prevention and control deficiencies cited in nursing homes during the pandemic

Narrative details	Month and year survey was conducted
State surveyors observed that high-touch surfaces were not being disinfected and that disinfecting supplies were not readily available for staff use. In addition, surveyors observed certified nursing assistants and a nurse in a nursing home not properly wearing personal protective equipment. Specifically, they observed these staff failing to change or properly wear personal protective equipment between residents with known or suspected COVID-19, such as two certified nursing assistants who did not change their gowns after providing care to a resident on droplet precautions. Two staff members indicated to surveyors that they had not been given any guidance on how long to wear personal protective equipment and when to change it.	July 2020
State surveyors observed staff members in a nursing home having direct contact with residents across both the COVID-19 negative and positive units. The surveyors also learned that the nursing home had not previously quarantined any residents after a known exposure to a COVID-19 positive roommate. In addition, surveyors learned that the infection preventionist continued to work in the facility and have direct contact with multiple residents in her role as a charge nurse after testing positive for COVID-19. She was immediately sent home after testing positive, but then she was directed to return to work the next day by the administration and continued to work her schedule. Further, surveyors observed challenges with personal protective equipment. They observed a certified nursing assistant provide personal care and assistance to several residents on the COVID-19 positive unit wearing a jumpsuit, instead of a gown, that she did not change between residents. She told the surveyors that she had been provided with the jumpsuit by the home and had been wearing it for several days. She did not remove the jumpsuit prior to leaving the nursing home at the end of her shift and would instead remove it on her porch and leave it there until her next shift. Then, she would clean it with disinfecting spray before putting it back on and returning to the home for her shift.	Sept. 2020

Narrative details	Month and year survey was conducted
State surveyors observed newly admitted residents were not being quarantined from other residents at a nursing home because, according to the Director of Nursing, there were challenges with space at the home. In addition, staff failed to properly use full personal protective equipment. The surveyors observed a certified nursing assistant coming out of a resident's room with her facemask around her chin and wearing eyeglasses with no face shield or goggles.	Feb. 2021
State surveyors observed certified nursing assistants in a nursing home assisting residents without performing any hand hygiene between residents. One certified nursing assistant was observed assisting a resident with adjusting a wheelchair and a bed side table. Then, she removed the resident's slice of bread from its wrapping with her bare hands and spread butter on the bread without performing any hand hygiene. Another certified nursing assistant did not perform hand hygiene when passing out lunch trays and setting up tray tables between residents. The certified nursing assistant said that she knew she should wash her hands between residents but she was trying to pass out the trays faster.	April 2021

Source: GAO analysis of Form-2567 deficiency narrative reports from the Centers for Medicare & Medicaid Services (CMS). | GAO-22-105133.

Appendix III: Types of Surveys and Investigations to Assess Whether Nursing Homes Are Meeting Federal Standards

As previously described, the Centers for Medicare & Medicaid Services (CMS) monitors nursing home compliance with federal standards primarily through the comprehensive standard surveys and as-needed investigations state survey agencies conduct. Beginning in March 2020, CMS required state survey agencies to conduct focused infection control surveys, a new type of survey developed by CMS and the Centers for Disease Control and Prevention (CDC) in response to the pandemic with a narrower scope than a standard survey. Focused infection control surveys assess federal standards for nursing home infection prevention and control that could contribute to the transmission of COVID-19, such as standards for personal protective equipment, testing, and isolating positive cases. CMS also suspended standard surveys and low priority investigations to limit surveyor time on site and focus state survey agency resources on limiting the spread of COVID-19.[74] Initially, state survey agencies conducted the focused infection control surveys in nursing homes specifically identified by HHS, and, beginning in June 2020, state survey agencies were required to conduct the focused infection control surveys any time a nursing home experienced a new COVID-19 outbreak.[75] Beginning in August 2020, CMS indicated state survey agencies should resume standard surveys as soon as they have the resources to conduct the surveys but also required them to continue conducting focused infection control surveys.[76] In January 2021 and again in November 2021, CMS changed the requirement for when a focused infection control survey must be conducted. Specifically, in November 2021, CMS required state survey agencies to perform focused infection control surveys for 20 percent of nursing homes in their state annually, prioritizing those facilities that report new COVID-19 cases and low vaccination rates, in addition to continuing to conduct standard surveys and investigations.[77] See figure 4 for a description of the types of surveys and investigations used to assess whether nursing homes are meeting federal standards as of April 2022.

---

[74] Under section 1135 of the Social Security Act, the Secretary of the Department of Health and Human Services (HHS) may temporarily waive or modify certain federal health care requirements, including those relating to standard surveys of nursing homes, when both a public health emergency and a disaster or emergency have been declared. 42 U.S.C. § 1320b-5. This authority was triggered on March 13, 2020, when the President declared the COVID-19 outbreak to be a national emergency under the National Emergencies Act and a nationwide emergency under section 501(b) of the Robert T. Stafford Disaster Relief and Emergency Assistance Act. The Secretary of HHS had previously declared COVID-19 a public health emergency on January 31, 2020, retroactive to January 27, 2020. See Centers for Medicare & Medicaid Services, QSO-20-20-ALL (March 20, 2020).

[75] CMS also required state survey agencies to conduct focused infection control surveys in all the nursing homes in their states by July 31, 2020 and in 20 percent of nursing homes in their states starting in fiscal year 2021. CMS also authorized states to expand certain survey activities, including standard surveys and high-priority complaint surveys, at the state's discretion. See Centers for Medicare & Medicaid Services, QSO-20-31-ALL (June 1, 2020) and Centers for Medicare & Medicaid Services, QSO-20-20-ALL (March 20, 2020).

[76] See Centers for Medicare & Medicaid Services, Enforcement Cases Held During the Prioritization Period and Revised Survey Prioritization, QSO-20-35-ALL (Baltimore, Md.: August 17, 2020).

[77] On November 30, 2020, elements of the focused infection control survey were incorporated into the standard survey process, in addition to maintaining the focused infection control survey as a stand-alone tool. See Centers for Medicare & Medicaid Services, QSO-20-31-ALL (January 4, 2021 revision) Also see Centers for Medicare & Medicaid Services, QSO-22-02-ALL (Nov. 12, 2021).

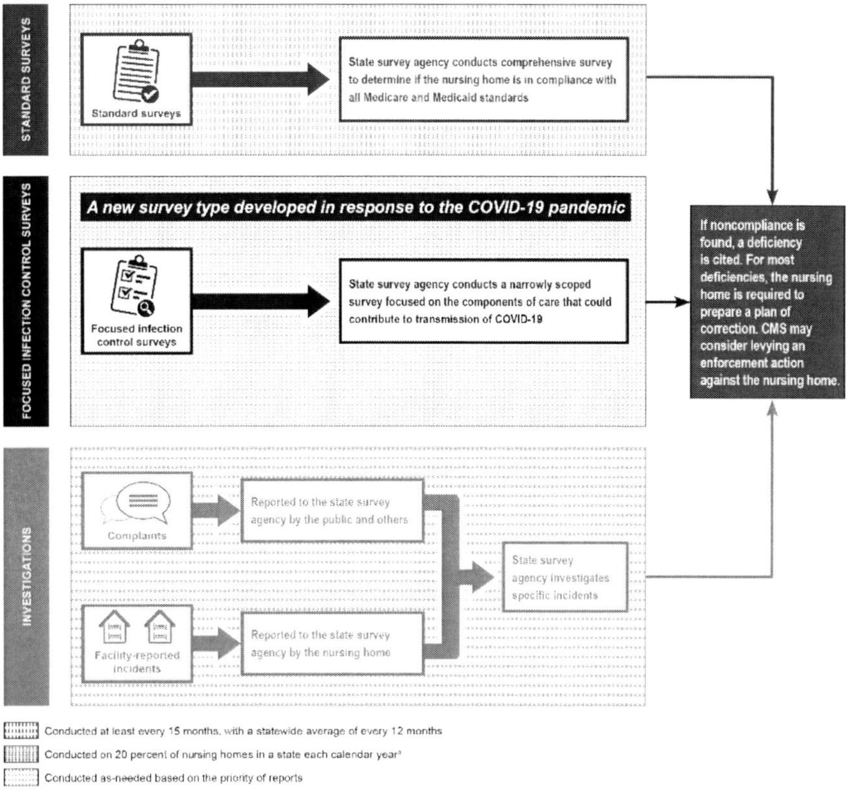

Source: GAO analysis of Centers for Medicare and Medicaid Services (CMS) data. | GAO-22-105133.

[a] Initially, state survey agencies conducted the focused infection control surveys in nursing homes specifically identified by the Department of Health and Human Services, and beginning in June 2020, state survey agencies were required to conduct the focused infection control surveys any time a nursing home experienced a new COVID-19 outbreak. Beginning in August 2020, CMS indicated state survey agencies should resume standard surveys as soon as they have the resources to conduct the surveys but also required them to continue conducting focused infection control surveys. In January 2021 and again in November 2021, CMS changed the requirement for when a focused infection control survey must be conducted. Specifically, in November 2021, CMS required state survey agencies to perform focused infection control surveys for 20 percent of nursing homes in their state annually, prioritizing those facilities that report new COVID-19 cases and low vaccination rates, in addition to continuing to conduct standard surveys and investigations.

Figure 4. Types of surveys and investigations used by state survey agencies to assess whether nursing homes are meeting federal standards, as of April 2022.

Appendix IV: Number and Percentage of Surveyed Nursing Homes with Infection Prevention and Control (IPC) Deficiencies

Table 3. Number and percentage of surveyed nursing homes with Infection Prevention and Control (IPC) deficiencies, by calendar year and deficiency code

2018	2019	2020		2021
Deficiency codes that went into effect prior to the pandemic				
F-880: IPC program[a]	6,316 (43.3%)	6,283 (42.5%)	6,810 (44.2%)	5,265 (37.3%)
F-881: Antibiotic stewardship program[b]	698 (4.8)	739 (5)	195 (1.3)	307 (2.2)
F-882: Infection preventionist role[c]	n/a	n/a	138 (0.9)	240 (1.7)
F-883: Influenza and pneumococcal immunization[d]	564 (3.9)	643 (4.4)	269 (1.7)	597 (4.2)
F-945: Infection control training[e]	n/a	n/a	n/a	n/a
F-884: Reporting to the National Healthcare Safety Network[f]	n/a	n/a	1,811 (11.8)	4,702 (33.3)
F-885: Reporting to residents, representatives, and families[g]	n/a	n/a	335 (2.2)	274 (1.9)
F-886: COVID-19 testing for residents and staff[h]	n/a	n/a	424 (2.8)	576 (4.1)
F-887: COVID-19 immunizations[i]	n/a	n/a	n/a	158 (1.1)
Total surveyed nursing homes	14,591	14,773	15,406	14,128

Source: GAO analysis of Centers for Medicare & Medicaid Services' (CMS) data. | GAO-22-105133.

[a] F-880 is the deficiency code for not meeting federal standards for establishing and maintaining an IPC program. This code went into effect as part of CMS's restructuring of its deficiency codes on November 28, 2017, replacing a prior deficiency code that had been in effect for several years.

[b] F-881 is the deficiency code for not meeting federal standards for establishing an effective antibiotic stewardship program. This deficiency code went into effect on November 28, 2017.

[c] F-882 is the deficiency code for not meeting federal standards for designating an infection preventionist. This deficiency code went into effect on November 28, 2019. State survey agencies began surveying nursing homes on it beginning August 26, 2020.

[d] F-883 is the deficiency code for not meeting federal standards for influenza and pneumococcal immunizations. This deficiency code went into effect as part of CMS's restructuring of its deficiency codes on November 28, 2017, replacing a prior deficiency code that had been in effect for several years.

[e] F-945 is the deficiency code for not meeting federal standards for infection control training. This deficiency code went into effect on November 28, 2019, but, at the time of our review, CMS had not yet directed state survey agencies to begin surveying homes on it. In June 2022, CMS announced that state survey agencies should begin surveying homes on this deficiency code beginning October 2022.

[f] F-884 is a COVID-19-specific deficiency code for not meeting federal standards for weekly COVID-19 reporting to the National Healthcare Safety Network. This deficiency code went into effect on May 6, 2020. Review for F-884 is conducted off-site by federal surveyors, who automatically cite nursing homes for not submitting timely and complete data of all reporting elements.

[g] F-885 is a COVID-19-specific deficiency code for not meeting federal standards for reporting COVID-19 cases to residents, representatives, and family. This deficiency code went into effect on May 6, 2020.

[h] F-886 is a COVID-19-specific deficiency code for not meeting federal standards for COVID-19 testing for residents and staff. This deficiency code went into effect on August 26, 2020.

[I] F-887 is a COVID-19 specific deficiency code for not meeting federal standards for COVID-19 immunizations. This deficiency code went into effect on May 11, 2021.

Appendix V: Federal Nursing Home Infection Prevention and Control (IPC) Actions

Table 4. Nursing Home Infection Prevention and Control (IPC) actions taken by the Centers for Medicare & Medicaid Services (CMS) and the Centers for Disease Control and Prevention (CDC)

Date	Action
Actions prior to the pandemic	
2009	CDC helped develop the *National Action Plan to Prevent Healthcare-Associated Infections: Roadmap to Elimination*, a plan intended to coordinate and maximize the efficiency of healthcare-associated infection prevention efforts across the federal government.[a]

Table 4. (Continued)

Date	Action
Actions prior to the pandemic	
	CDC began working with state-based Healthcare-Associated Infection programs, which are able to provide on-the-ground IPC assessments and technical assistance in nursing homes and other health care facilities.
2012	CDC created a module in the National Healthcare Safety Network for national infection surveillance that allowed nursing homes to voluntarily report infections, such as *C. difficile*. [b] CDC conducted the National Survey of Long-Term Care Providers to collect information from nursing homes on IPC practices, as well as the immunization status of and infection burden among nursing home residents. CMS begins to publicly report influenza and pneumococcal vaccination of nursing home residents and other IPC quality measures, such as urinary tract infections among residents.
2015	CDC developed and released the Core Elements of Antibiotic Stewardship for Nursing Homes which outlines steps nursing homes and other long-term care facilities could take to improve antibiotic prescribing practices and reduce their inappropriate use.
2016	CDC developed and released an IPC assessment tool to assist health departments and facilities assess infection control programs and practices in nursing homes and other long-term care facilities. [c] CMS published a final rule revising requirements for nursing homes' broader IPC program with varying implementation dates. The requirements implemented in 2016 included that nursing homes must have a system for preventing, identifying, reporting, investigating, and controlling infections and communicable diseases for residents and staff. [d]
2017	CMS required nursing homes to develop an antibiotic stewardship program to combat the growing concern of multi-drug resistant organisms. [e]
2019	CMS and CDC collaborated on the development of a free on-line infection preventionist training course. [f] CMS and CDC released the Nursing Home Infection Control Worksheet, a nursing home self-assessment tool developed through a 3-year pilot program across 40 participating nursing homes. CMS required nursing homes to designate an infection preventionist who works at least part-time at the facility. CMS updated surveyor interpretive guidance to clarify that a facility's emergency preparedness planning should include "emerging infectious diseases."

Date	Action
Actions during the pandemic	
Feb. 14, 2020	CMS created and released the "Head to Toe Toolkit," offering educational materials and interventions for bedside staff to prevent common infections.
Starting on Feb. 27, 2020	CDC conducted about 100 COVID-19 outbreak investigations in nursing homes and other long-term care facilities in collaboration with local and state health departments. [g]
Mar. 1, 2020	CDC issued guidance to assist nursing homes' response to COVID-19. [h] CMS initiated blanket waivers to grant nursing homes flexibilities, such as waiving certain training and certification requirements for certified nurse aides.
Mar. 4, 2020	CMS prioritized certain survey activities, such as surveys responding to allegations of abuse and neglect.
Mar. 13, 2020	CMS restricted all visitors and non-essential health care personnel from entering nursing homes, with exceptions made for compassionate care situations, such as end-of-life situations. Surveyors were also granted access. Cancelled communal dining and group activities.
Mar. 20, 2020	CMS temporarily suspended all standard surveys and suspended some other types of survey work. CMS released a targeted IPC survey tool—the focused infection control survey—and instructed states to use this survey in place of the standard survey process. CMS suspended most enforcement actions for facilities not in substantial compliance, until revisit surveys could be resumed.
May 6, 2020	CMS created new deficiency codes, known as F-tags (F-884 and F-885) associated with required reporting of cases and deaths to CDC through the National Healthcare Safety Network and to residents, their representatives, and their families.
June 1, 2020	CMS initiated a performance-based funding requirement tying CARES Act supplemental grants for state survey agencies to the completion of focused infection control surveys. CMS increased penalties for noncompliance with IPC, making the penalties more significant for those nursing homes with a history of past IPC deficiencies or that caused actual harm to residents or immediate jeopardy. CMS announced the deployment of Quality Improvement Organizations to provide technical assistance to approximately 3,000 low-performing nursing homes that had a history of IPC challenges.
June 4, 2020	CMS announced it will post survey results that were conducted on or after March 4, 2020 on Nursing Home Compare.

Table 4. (Continued)

Date	Action
June 23 through Aug. 19, 2020	CMS convened the Coronavirus Commission for Safety and Quality in Nursing Homes, a committee of experts tasked to identify lessons learned from the early days of the pandemic and develop recommendations for future actions to improve IPC measures in nursing homes. [i]
July 18, 2020	The Department of Health and Human Services (HHS), including CDC and CMS staff, began sending strike teams to nursing homes to assist with responding to COVID-19 outbreaks.
Aug. 17, 2020	CMS authorized the resumption of standard surveys.
Aug. 25, 2020	CMS released a national nursing home training program for frontline staff and management.
Aug. 26, 2020	CMS set civil monetary penalties for failure to report COVID-related data to the National Healthcare Safety Network, associated with any F-884 citation.
Aug. 26, 2020	CMS created a new F-tag (F-886) associated with required COVID-19 testing of nursing homes staff and residents and proper documentation of testing data. CMS updated the focused infection control survey tool to assess compliance with new COVID-19 testing requirements, as well as prior updates in guidance. CMS temporarily updated the focused infection control survey tool to assess compliance with the requirement to designate an infection preventionist.
Sept. 17, 2020	CMS changed restrictions on nursing home visitation to allow limited indoor visits while still adhering to social distancing precautions. [j]
Oct. 29, 2020	CDC launched the Project Firstline Healthcare Infection Control Training Collaborative, a coalition of health care, public health, and academic partners who developed interactive infection control trainings for all health care workers, including nursing home staff.
Nov. 30, 2020	CMS integrated elements of the focused infection control survey tool into the standard survey IPC pathway for all standard surveys beginning after November 30, 2020, in addition to maintaining the focused infection control survey as a stand-alone tool.
Dec. 4, 2020	CMS announced the agency will resume calculating nursing home health inspection and quality measure ratings on January 27, 2021.
Dec. 21, 2020	CDC launched the federal Pharmacy Partnership for Long-term Care program to bring COVID-19 vaccine clinics to residents and staff members in nursing homes across the country.

Date	Action
Jan. 4, 2021	CMS revised the criteria requiring states to conduct focused infection control surveys.
Mar. 10, 2021	CMS further changed some visitation restrictions by allowing visitation even when a nursing home had COVID-19 positive residents and permitting physical contact between visitors and residents when a resident is vaccinated.
May 11, 2021	CMS published an interim final rule that established requirements regarding offering COVID-19 vaccines to residents and staff and established an accompanying new F-tag (F-887). CMS also began requiring the reporting of vaccination data to CDC. [k]
Oct. 1, 2021	CDC, in partnership with CMS, provided funding for state-based strike teams to provide surge capacity, address staffing shortages, and strengthen IPC activities in nursing homes. [l]
Nov. 12, 2021	CMS announced steps to assist state survey agencies in addressing the backlog of complaint and standard surveys. These steps included revising the criteria for conducting a focused infection control survey so that a survey is not required in response to COVID-19 outbreaks and providing guidance for resuming standard surveys.
Nov. 12, 2021	CMS began allowing nursing home visitation for all residents at all times.
Dec. 28, 2021	CMS began issuing guidance requiring health care staff vaccination. Additional guidance was released in January 2022.
April 7, 2022	CMS announced plans to phase in an end to certain emergency declaration blanket waivers for nursing homes, such as the waiver allowing nursing homes to employ nurse aides that have not completed a full course of training, which would end on June 6, 2022. [m]

Source: GAO summary of CMS and CDC identified actions. | GAO-22-105133.

[a] In 2013, the Department of Health and Human Services released an update to the National Action Plan that included a chapter on healthcare-associated infection prevention across the long-term care spectrum, including in nursing homes. Department of Health and Human Services, The National Action Plan to Prevent Health Care-Associated Infections: Road Map to Elimination (Washington, D.C.: 2013).

[b] Between 2016 and 2018, CDC, CMS, and a network of health care quality improvement organizations enrolled 2,000 nursing homes in the National Healthcare Safety Network to report and track C. difficile bacterial infections in order to support antibiotic stewardship and infection prevention practices. C. difficile is a bacterium that causes severe diarrhea and inflammation of the colon and infections result in disproportionately higher rates of hospitalization and death in individuals over the age of 65. During the pandemic, CDC expanded the National Health Care Safety Network to allow for reporting of COVID-19 cases and deaths from nursing homes, as well as other COVID-19 related data such as nursing home access to testing, personal protective supplies, and staff and resident vaccinations.

[c] The IPC assessment for nursing homes–known as the Infection Control Assessment and Response tool–was later adapted and used by health departments and other partners to perform remote video-assisted or onsite assessment of COVID-19-specific IPC practices and guide quality improvement activities in nursing homes.

[d] Medicare and Medicaid Programs; Reform of Requirements for Long-Term Care Facilities, 81 Fed. Reg. 68,688 (Oct. 4, 2016).

[e] CDC also implemented initiatives to address antibiotic-resistant infections and to promote antibiotic stewardship efforts in nursing homes to align with CDC's activities to address antibiotic resistance as outlined in the U.S. National Action Plan for Combating Antibiotic -Resistant Bacteria, which was issued in 2015. See The White House, U.S. National Action Plan for Combating Antibiotic-Resistant Bacteria (Washington, D.C.: March 2015).

[f] CMS also created a nursing home antibiotic stewardship program training.

[g] CDC has provided further outbreak investigation and support services. For example, according to CDC officials, the CDC funded Healthcare-Associated Infection and Antimicrobial Resistance Prevention Programs that assisted with over 21,000 COVID-19 outbreak investigations in nursing homes. CDC staff along with state and local health departments also conducted thousands of Infection Control Assessment and Response assessments (both in-person and by telephone) in long-term care facilities, including nursing homes.

[h] Specifically, on March 1, 2020, CDC issued Responding to COVID-19 in Nursing Homes and Performing Facility-wide SARS-CoV-2 Testing in Nursing Homes, as a supplemental addition to CDC's overall IPC guidance, initially released January 28, 2020. The nursing home-specific guidance was updated multiple times during the pandemic. In addition, on March 17, 2020, CDC began a series of clinician outreach and communication activity calls on COVID-19 in nursing homes and other long-term care facilities. See Centers for Disease Control and Prevention, Interim Infection Prevention and Control Recommendations to Prevent SARS-CoV-2 Spread in Nursing Homes, accessed on November 8, 2021, https://www.cdc.gov/coronavirus/2019-ncov/hcp/long-term-care.html. This online guidance was merged with Centers for Disease Control and Prevention, responding to COVID-19 in Nursing Homes and Centers for Disease Control and Prevention, Performing Facility-wide SARS-CoV-2 Testing in Nursing Homes, as of March 29, 2021.

[i] The Commission's final report was issued in September 2020. MITRE, Coronavirus Commission on Safety and Quality in Nursing Homes, Commission Final Report (McLean, Va.: The MITRE Corporation, 2020). This report was written for CMS under a government contract.

[j] CMS also changed restrictions on communal activities and dining.

[k] Medicare and Medicaid Programs; COVID-19 Vaccine Requirements for Long-Term Care Facilities and Intermediate Care Facilities for Individuals with Intellectual Disabilities Residents, Clients, and Staff, 86 Fed. Reg. 26,306, 26,336 (May 13, 2021).

[l] The purpose of the funding is to assist nursing homes during their response to COVID-19 infections, and to build and maintain the infection prevention infrastructure necessary to support resident, visitor, and facility healthcare personnel safety. According to CDC officials, funding to health departments to conduct these activities has been distributed and CDC continues to provide technical expertise and assistance to the recipients.

[m] CMS had previously waived the requirement that nursing homes may not employ anyone for longer than four months unless they met the training and certification requirements under section 483.35(d) of title 42 of the Code of Federal Regulations.

Appendix VI: Comments from the Department of Health and Human Services

DEPARTMENT OF HEALTH & HUMAN SERVICES

OFFICE OF THE SECRETARY

Assistant Secretary for Legislation
Washington, DC 20201

July 26, 2022

John E. Dicken
Director, Health Care
U.S. Government Accountability Office
441 G Street NW
Washington, DC 20548

Dear Mr. Dicken:

Attached are comments on the U.S. Government Accountability Office's (GAO) report entitled, **"COVID-19 IN NURSING HOMES: CMS Needs to Continue to Strengthen Oversight of Infection Prevention and Control"** (GAO-22-105133).

The Department appreciates the opportunity to review this report prior to publication.

Sincerely,

Melanie Anne Egorin

Melanie Anne Egorin, PhD
Assistant Secretary for Legislation

Attachment

GENERAL COMMENTS FROM THE DEPARTMENT OF HEALTH AND HUMAN SERVICES ON THE GOVERNMENT ACCOUNTABILITY OFFICE'S DRAFT REPORT ENTITLED - COVID-19 IN NURSING HOMES: CMS NEEDS TO CONTINUE TO STRENGTHEN OVERSIGHT OF INFECTION PREVENTION AND CONTROL (GAO-22-105133)

The Department of Health & Human Services (HHS) appreciates the opportunity to review and comment on the Government Accountability Office's (GAO) draft report.

General Comments

The Centers for Medicare & Medicaid Services (CMS) takes seriously its role in improving the safety and quality of care in our nation's nursing homes, and as such, CMS is leading the Biden-Harris Administration's new efforts to increase accountability for nursing homes. The Administration has laid out 21 initiatives spread across five key strategic goals, including a goal to ensure pandemic and emergency preparedness in nursing homes and carry forward lessons learned during the COVID-19 public health emergency.[1] These initiatives were developed with extensive input from advocates, industry experts, nursing home workers, and most importantly, residents and their loved ones. CMS is considering a wide range of methods to accomplish this important work.

Nursing homes receiving Medicare or Medicaid payments are required to comply with CMS quality and safety standards, including those relating to infection prevention and control and emergency preparedness. CMS shares management of nursing home oversight with State Survey Agencies (SSAs) who conduct onsite surveys to assess compliance with the Federal requirements and investigate facility complaints. SSAs serve as the front-line responders to address health and safety concerns raised by residents, their families, and facility staff. Accordingly, when an SSA identifies an issue of non-compliance, the nursing home is cited for a deficiency and is required to correct the issue(s) and demonstrate substantial compliance with all Federal requirements.

Long before the COVID-19 pandemic began, CMS had acted to strengthen infection prevention and control practices in nursing homes. CMS took pivotal actions in the 2016 final rule, Emergency Preparedness Requirements for Medicare and Medicaid Participating Providers and Suppliers, which outlined the need for nursing homes to prepare for infectious disease threats.[2] CMS also outlined specific reform requirements for long-term care (LTC) facilities in the 2016 final rule, Medicare and Medicaid Programs: Reform of Requirements for Long-Term Care Facilities, which was the impetus for the requirement that nursing homes develop an infection prevention and control program that includes an antibiotic stewardship program.[3]

Since the COVID-19 public health emergency declaration in early 2020, CMS has taken a number of actions to further strengthen infection prevention and control within nursing homes. CMS began by issuing guidance to nursing homes encouraging them to take appropriate action to address potential and confirmed COVID-19 cases and mitigate transmission. CMS reiterated the importance of longstanding infection control guidelines, and guidelines on screening processes and the use of personal protective equipment. CMS has held regular calls with stakeholders, nursing home associations, and State Agencies to keep them up to date on the latest information to respond to COVID-19. Through the Quality Improvement Organizations (QIOs) CMS also sent federal strike teams comprised of representatives from Centers for Disease Control and

[1] The White House, FACT SHEET: Protecting Seniors by Improving Safety and Quality of Care in the Nation's Nursing Homes, February 28, 2022.

[2] Medicare and Medicaid Programs, Emergency Preparedness Requirements, 81 Fed. Reg. 63860, 63862 (Sept. 16, 2016).

[3] Medicare and Medicaid Programs; Reform of Requirements for Long-Term Care Facilities, 81 Fed. Reg. 68688 (Nov. 28, 2016).

GENERAL COMMENTS FROM THE DEPARTMENT OF HEALTH AND HUMAN SERVICES ON THE GOVERNMENT ACCOUNTABILITY OFFICE'S DRAFT REPORT ENTITLED - COVID-19 IN NURSING HOMES: CMS NEEDS TO CONTINUE TO STRENGTHEN OVERSIGHT OF INFECTION PREVENTION AND CONTROL (GAO-22-105133)

Prevention (CDC), CMS, and the Office of the Assistant Secretary for Health (OASH) to help facilities address COVID-19 challenges related to staffing, personal protective equipment supplies, COVID-19 testing, and infection prevention and control measure implementation.

In an effort to focus on controlling the spread of COVID-19, CMS provided SSAs with a streamlined review tool to conduct focused infection control surveys of providers identified through collaboration with the CDC and the Assistant Secretary for Preparedness and Response (ASPR). This tool was shared with providers who were encouraged by CMS to use it to self-assess their own ability to prevent the spread of COVID-19. By July 2020, over 99 percent of nursing homes had a focused infection control survey conducted onsite. As the public health emergency continued, the focused infection control survey was revised to incorporate new infection control requirements to address the spread of COVID-19. While the COVID-19 public health emergency warranted a more targeted approach for assessing a nursing homes' compliance with infection prevention and control requirements, in November 2021, CMS released a memorandum on Changes to COVID-19 Survey Activities and Increased Oversight in Nursing Homes to help SSAs focus their efforts on identifying concerns for all aspects of quality of care, quality of life, and ensuring health and safety.[4] CMS now requires SSAs to perform annual focused infection control surveys at 20 percent of nursing homes.[5] CMS also published a toolkit comprised of recommendations and best practices from a variety of frontline health care providers, state governors' COVID-19 task forces, associations, and other experts that is intended to serve as a catalogue of resources dedicated to addressing the specific challenges facing nursing homes as they combat COVID-19.[6] CMS continues to review and revise guidance as appropriate.

In addition to the survey process used to verify compliance with Federal requirements, CMS uses data submitted by nursing homes to improve oversight and inform the public. CMS implemented a requirement that Medicare-certified nursing homes report COVID-19 testing, case, and mortality data for residents and staff to the CDC's National Healthcare Safety Network.[7] Thereafter, in September of 2021, CMS began posting nursing home staff and resident COVID-19 vaccination data in a user-friendly format on its Nursing Home Care Compare website. Subsequently, in February 2022, CMS began posting staff and resident booster shot data to the website.[8] To further enhance the information available to consumers, residents, and families and to help support their healthcare decisions and incentivize quality improvement among nursing homes, CMS began posting weekend nurse staffing levels as well as nursing home staff turnover data.[9]

These data are also used in the coordinated effort between CMS and CDC to provide detailed information to state and local health departments and nursing homes to inform infection

[4] QSO-22-02-All: Changes to COVID-19 Survey Activities and Increased Oversight in Nursing Homes.
[5] QSO-22-02-All: Changes to COVID-19 Survey Activities and Increased Oversight in Nursing Homes.
[6] QSO-21-08-NLTC: COVID-19 Focused Infection Control Survey Tool for Acute and Continuing Care Providers and Suppliers.
[7] QSO-20-26-NH Upcoming Requirements for Notification of Confirmed COVID-19 (or COVID-19 Persons under Investigation) Among Residents and Staff in Nursing Homes.
[8] CMS Makes Nursing Home COVID-19 Booster Vaccination Online Increasing Transparency, CMS News Alert, Feb. 09, 2022.
[9] QSO-22-0-08-NH: Nursing Home Staff Turnover and Weekend Staffing Levels.

GENERAL COMMENTS FROM THE DEPARTMENT OF HEALTH AND HUMAN SERVICES ON THE GOVERNMENT ACCOUNTABILITY OFFICE'S DRAFT REPORT ENTITLED - COVID-19 IN NURSING HOMES: CMS NEEDS TO CONTINUE TO STRENGTHEN OVERSIGHT OF INFECTION PREVENTION AND CONTROL (GAO-22-105133)

prevention and control policies and strategies across the country to further support nursing home residents. These data are also used by CMS when it is considering adjusting or introducing new policies. They have informed CMS's national policies as to when to implement, revise, or terminate waivers, and they have allowed CMS to target specific nursing homes for assistance with infection control or vaccine uptake. Specifically, through the work of the Quality Improvement Organization (QIO) program, CMS assists nursing homes in strengthening infection control practices to reduce and prevent transmission of COVID-19.

The QIOs provide educational activities, including frontline training of nursing home staff and management on infection prevention practices to reduce the spread of infection and manage outbreaks effectively, as well as providing individualized training resources based on the nursing homes' specific needs through toolkits, resource materials, guides, webinars, and clinician office hours to provide expert consultation on the particular challenges nursing homes face. CMS collects best practices and lessons learned from each of the QIOs and coordinates the sharing of that information across QIOs nationally for rapid deployment. Additionally, CMS partners with Federal agencies such as the CDC and ASPR, who are the national leaders in disease prevention and control and public health emergency response to ensure coordination of services and alignment of guidance for nursing homes.

As we continue to emerge from the COVID-19 pandemic, ensuring that residents in nursing home receive safe, high-quality care is critical. CMS is continuing the work it started before the COVID-19 pandemic to strengthen its health and safety requirements that protect residents' rights and improve the quality of care they receive. Based on lessons learned from the pandemic, CMS released guidance related to the requirement for all nursing homes to have an Infection Preventionist (IP) who has specialized training to effectively oversee the facility's infection prevention and control program. With emerging infectious disease such as COVID-19, CMS believes the role of the IP is critical in nursing homes' efforts to mitigate the onset and spread of infections. CMS recently revised guidance to clarify its expectations for infection control and prevention.[10]

HHS and CMS thank GAO for its efforts on this important issue and look forward to working with GAO on this and other issues in the future. GAO's recommendations and CMS' responses are below.

GAO Recommendation 1
Establish minimum infection preventionist training standards.

HHS Response
CMS concurs with this recommendation. CMS will consider this recommendation when proposing new requirements. We note that any proposed regulation requires notice and comment rulemaking. Currently, the regulation at 42 C.F.R. § 483.80(b) states that the IP who is responsible for the facility's infection prevention and control program must 1) have primary

[10] QSO-22-19-NH Revised Long-Term Care Surveyor Guidance: Revisions to Surveyor Guidance for Phase 2 & 3, Arbitration Agreement Requirements, Investigating Complaints & Facility Reported Incidents, and the Psychosocial Outcome Severity Guide.

GENERAL COMMENTS FROM THE DEPARTMENT OF HEALTH AND HUMAN SERVICES ON THE GOVERNMENT ACCOUNTABILITY OFFICE'S DRAFT REPORT ENTITLED - COVID-19 IN NURSING HOMES: CMS NEEDS TO CONTINUE TO STRENGTHEN OVERSIGHT OF INFECTION PREVENTION AND CONTROL (GAO-22-105133)

professional training in nursing, medical technology, microbiology, epidemiology, or another related field; 2) be qualified by education, training, experience or certification; 3) have completed specialized training in infection prevention and control.[11] Additionally, CDC and CMS developed specialized IP training to include topics such as transmission based precautions and antibiotic stewardship programs.[12] While CMS does not dictate which specialized training in infection prevention and control is required, the IP would be expected to have completed specialized training prior to being hired or being designated as an IP.

GAO Recommendation 2
Collect infection preventionist staffing data and use these data to determine whether the current infection preventionist staffing requirement is sufficient.

HHS Response
CMS will consider this recommendation when proposing new requirements. We note that any proposed regulation requires notice and comment rulemaking. CMS recently revised guidance for implementing Phase 3 regulations, among which requires nursing homes to have an IP who has specialized training onsite at least part-time to effectively oversee the facility's infection prevention and control program.[13] With emerging infectious diseases such as COVID-19, CMS believes the role of the IP is critical in a facility's efforts to mitigate the onset and spread of infections. Currently, the regulation at 42 C.F.R. § 483.70(f) states all LTC facilities are responsible for employing full-time, part-time, or on a consultant basis those professionals necessary to carry out the provisions of the LTC requirements.[14] Thus, LTC facilities are currently required to have *at least* a part-time IP, which should be seen as a minimum for LTC facilities needing an IP for a longer time, as the IP must meet the needs of the facility. SSAs are responsible for ensuring nursing homes are complying with this and other Federal requirements.

Further, the current regulation at 42 C.F.R. § 483.70 requires LTC facilities to submit complete and accurate direct care staffing information, including information for agency and contract staff, based on payroll and other verifiable and auditable data, which is currently done through the Electronic Staffing Data Submission Payroll-Based Journal.[15] CMS must consider the ability to audit the staffing data in order to be consistent with the statutory requirement. CMS will evaluate the feasibility of collecting this information, and will take appropriate actions based on this evaluation.

GAO Recommendation 3
Provide additional guidance in the State Operations Manual on making scope and severity determination for IPC-related deficiencies

[11] *See also*, Medicare and Medicaid Programs; Reform of Requirements for Long-Term Care Facilities, 81 Fed. Reg. 68688 (Nov. 28, 2016).
[12] CDC Train, Nursing Home Infection Preventionist Training Course.
[13] QSO-22-19-NH Revised Long-Term Care Surveyor Guidance: Revisions to Surveyor Guidance for Phase 2 & 3, Arbitration Agreement Requirements, Investigating Complaints & Facility Reported Incidents, and the Psychosocial Outcome Severity Guide.
[14] Requirements for States and Long-Term Care Facilities, 42 CFR Part 483.70.
[15] S&C: 17-45-NH Electronic Staffing Submission - Payroll-Based Journal (PBJ)

GENERAL COMMENTS FROM THE DEPARTMENT OF HEALTH & HUMAN SERVICES ON THE GOVERNMENT ACCOUNTABILITY OFFICE'S DRAFT REPORT ENTITLED - COVID-19 IN NURSING HOMES: CMS NEEDS TO CONTINUE TO STRENGTHEN OVERSIGHT OF INFECTION PREVENTION AND CONTROL (GAO-22-105133)

HHS Response

In June 2022, CMS updated Appendix PP of the State Operations Manual to, among other things, provide additional guidance for infection prevention and control (IPC)-related deficiencies.[16] The new guidance includes additional examples surveyors can use to assess the scope and severity of IPC-related deficiencies. For example, CMS provided deficiency categorization examples at each of the four severity levels for both the infection control deficiency F-880 and the infection preventionist deficiency F-883. Given this additional information, CMS believes it met the recommendation requirements prior to the report publication and requests that GAO remove this recommendation.

[16] QSO-22-19-NH Revised Long-Term Care Surveyor Guidance: Revisions to Surveyor Guidance for Phase 2 & 3, Arbitration Agreement Requirements, Investigating Complaints & Facility Reported Incidents, and the Psychosocial Outcome Severity Guide.

Index

N

O

P